Wildflowers and Wooden Spoons

Stories and Recipes from Mother Earth Cafe

Patricia Lucia

Noble Light Press

First Edition November 2021

Illustrations copyright © 2021 by Bridget Van Otteren

Cover Design © 2021 by Ashe Rodriguez

Food photography by Ashe Rodriguez

Author photo by Ashe Rodriguez

ISBN: 9780578873350

Published by Noble Light Press

noblelightpress.com

To Bridget, Taylor, Keahi and Kris

With so much love and gratitude

And to the late Terry Murphy

Chef, Mentor and Friend

Table of Contents

Introduction

Wildflowers and Wooden Spoons is the second in a three book series—with the first, *Wildflowers and Present Tenses* released in November 2020, and the next, *Wildflowers and Laughing Crones* projected for release in November of 2022. *Wildflowers and Wooden Spoons* departs from the structure of the first and last of this series as it is a cookbook. A Cookbook? And while I'm tempted to break into the *Sesame Street* song *"One of These Things is Not Like the Others"*, I think it best I explain the sequence of events which led to this odd placement of a cookbook.

At the beginning of 2020, I made a commitment to complete that book I'd been wanting to write for nearly twenty years. In fact, I had moved from apartment to apartment, and even from New York City to South Florida with the box of stories I had written while earning my Master's degree in Creative Writing at City College of New York. I had promised my professor I would write that collection and he had promised he would pick up a copy at Barnes and Noble. But then 9/11 happened, and I packed up my stories and my life and headed to Florida. I settled into a new life in Florida and a new teaching job, and within a few years, had opened a coffeehouse cafe, a longtime dream of mine. I began a new adventure, and, stepping away from my teaching career of nearly twenty years, devoted everything I had to keeping that little place going. And I did for nearly ten years. If you know anything about little coffeehouses and cafes, you know they are filled with magic and stories. Mother Earth Sanctuary Cafe was known for miles around and I was mostly called "Mother Earth" around town. When we closed our doors

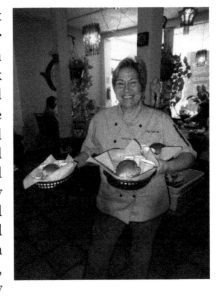

at the end of 2016, locals urged me to open again in another location, or get a food truck or cater. But for me, while the closing had initially felt like a heartbreak, it slowly began to feel like a relief. I was exhausted, depleted beyond what I had thought. I took some time for myself back in Massachusetts and when I came home to Florida again, I returned to teaching and to my writing again.

Wildflowers and Wooden Spoons is a much anticipated cookbook with all the signature recipes from Mother Earth Sanctuary Cafe. Recipes my former customers have been requesting for years. I have included stories from the cafe and some personal anecdotes to introduce many of the recipes. This collection, just like the cafe, has something for everyone, no matter what your eating preferences are. There are vegan, vegetarian, and meat dishes. I include suggestions for variations on recipes. For instance, one can make a vegan recipe a meat recipe or a meat recipe a vegan recipe. I do not cater to one group over the other, and have not marked which recipes are which. I admit I may have decided on that latter part just to be snarky.

So in 2020 when the lockdowns gave me plenty of time and opportunity to focus on my writing, I chose to complete the stories that had been waiting the longest, stories still tucked in the corner of the cardboard box in which they had traveled from New York City. These were raw, coming of age stories, coming out stories, love stories, heartbreak stories, and stories about a young woman searching for meaning. Stories about a woman who did not yet believe in her own magic. I needed to start there. *Wildflowers and Present Tenses* takes readers through time and drops them at the door of a little cafe. A Crone narrator - my future self - floats in and out between the stories as fairies listen and indulge in libation. The Crone returns again in this cookbook and the fairies flit around in the corners of pages.

If you have been waiting for cafe recipes, I thank you for your patience. I sincerely hope you enjoy the food, the stories and the magic, and that you stir plenty of your own magic into the orbit of your wooden spoons.

- Patti

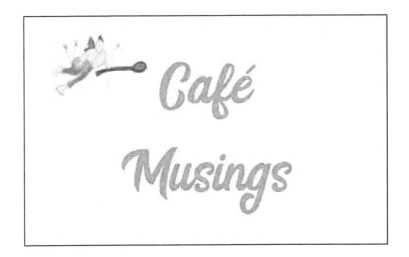

The Crone

The Crone stands at her sink with her hands in the warm dish water and looks out on the bright purples and yellows of wildflowers growing along the edges of her herb garden. Her fingers skim the sink for the last of her dishes. Like tea leaves on the bottom of a cup or a tarot card pulled to answer a question, the Crone finds doorways through time with the last utensil in her sink. She finds a wooden spoon floating in the suds and smiles at the sight of it in her hand. A small figure moves - perhaps a hummingbird or dragonfly - and lands on the windowsill in front of her and is still, listening.

Her thoughts travel back to a kitchen in a small cafe and further to the kitchen in her childhood home and still further back to a distant past when she held her first spoon, carved by her own hands. She glances up at her small, winged audience and tells her story.

The voices that whispered to me in that cafe kitchen, the voices I thought were spirits of ancestors or medicine women spirits in the mango tree - those voices were always me. The past me, the future me, all the versions of me.

The kitchen is the perfect place for such whispers. It is quiet except for the sound of food being prepared, chopped, stirred, sizzling, boiling. The aromas in the kitchen naturally unlock ancient memory, open portals to our past selves, stir past voices to speak into our ears. Most of the time I was not conscious of slipping into a meditative state. I became conscious of the whispers though, and was often surprised by what they said. It never occurred to me that the voices I heard could be my ancient selves smiling, laughing, chatting, instructing and critiquing what I was doing in that kitchen.

My growing love of spices from India and Africa. All me. Ancient versions of me, preparing food for family and tribe. Memories. I have fed so many for so very long. We all have. It is an essential part of our human journey and so a foundational memory tucked away in our marrow - DNA memories scientists do not yet understand. The concept of storing ancient memory from ancient lifetimes - soul memory - has no basis in modern science.

But when I stood in that tiny cafe kitchen, day after day making bread with my hands, stirring soup with wooden spoons, surrounded by the aroma of spices and herbs, the sounds of chopping and stirring, moving my hands in old familiar patterns, ancient memories deep in my marrow woke and flowed freely in my blood through my heart, through all of me. Spirits of the past rushed in. The kitchen was full and bustling, even when I was alone. And the chatter in the room was incessant.

What is she doing?

Something with sweet potato.

Oh! Then curry! Curry would be nice.

Cumin, too.

Cayenne for a little heat.

Recipes came quickly and naturally. It felt like magic. My young staff felt it. My customers felt it. None of us understood what was really going on. We felt a presence there and thought it was the spirits associated with that magnificent tree outside the kitchen door. I felt a sort of portal but understood the concept of energetic portals in narrow terms. I believed portals were connected to outer realms, not inner ones. That spirits were 'others', not aspects and versions of myself.

Art is a portal. I had discovered that with the colorful paintings I created and hung on the walls. When I became inspired to create art with the spices I used, the spice art created new portals to an ancient and vibrant past. Such deep, rich, beautiful colors, I had mused. The many hues of humans. Soon portraits of human ancestors occupied the cafe walls, inspired by the spices that brought their faces to life. I did not know the humans whose images I had 'painted 'with cinnamon and cumin and curry and chili, but they knew me. I had created portals to ancient aspects of myself, to ancient versions of all those who entered my cafe.

These memories come back to me whenever I stand in this humble kitchen as I do now, and lift the lid off a pot that has occupied my stove for hours. I mostly feed myself and my beloved these days, but my kitchen is still crowded and full of chatter on a day like today when I dote on a pot of soup or knead the dough for our daily herbed bread. The color of these spices still remind me of skin tones I have worn, and the aroma brings me back to those kitchens where my brown hands moved and turned flat breads on cast iron, skinned and cut up meat, and pounded spices into powder. The sound of animal fat sizzling and snapping transports me back to northern regions where my ruddy hands cut and cooked blubber in long strips like bacon.

And these hands have held wooden spoons in every corner of the world. I have called family and tribe in every tongue, beaconing them to the hearth and table. My soul will always be at home in the kitchen. And so it will be in the next when my future being picks up a wooden spoon and feels a mysterious sense of joy and curiosity. Ah, the first of many memories moving from my ancient future marrow to my heart. And there I will begin another dance in the kitchen.

Kitchen Magic

I experienced kitchen magic most intensely in my little cafe, Mother Earth Sanctuary Cafe—which had begun as a coffeehouse in March of 2007 and evolved into the cafe I ran until the end of 2016. In the early coffeehouse days, when it had the 'punny 'name of Les Beans Coffee, the magic of the place mostly happened on the small stage in the front of the house. Open Mic nights were most magical, drawing young musicians, poets and storytellers from all over the county on Thursdays nights. At the height of its

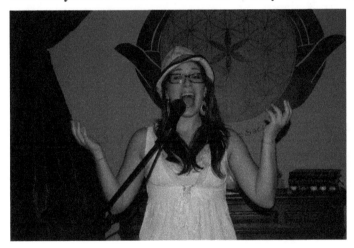

popularity, nearly one hundred people packed the cafe's 800 square foot area (apologies to the fire marshals) to support the creatives taking to the stage to share a song, poem or story. When I expanded the menu and evolved into a scratch kitchen cafe, the stage was replaced by tables to accommodate our busy lunches. I did not know it at the time, but the magic moved from the front of the house to the back of the house. The kitchen.

Often in the early hours of the day when I prepared food quietly, meditatively, new inspirations whispered in my ear. I believe this is the same state of grace artists experience when creating. A kind of quiet openness to unseen forces that inspire and help move a paint brush or pen, put new and unexpected ideas before us or in my case, whisper recipe ideas, herb and spice combinations that were outside my base of knowledge and experience. I pondered ancient ways of food preparation and the movement of energy through food.

Food preparation is engrained in our DNA memory. How many lifetimes have we baked bread or stirred a pot of soup? Could this be why our associations with bread and soup are so evocative and why we are so comforted by their aroma? I spent enough time in the kitchen to contemplate these things. I wondered how many times I had kneaded the dough for bread, made a pot of soup. How many souls had I fed? Then a thought occurred to me. I remembered that our oldest memories are carried through our sense of smell. Aromas transport us to other places. Memories older perhaps than this life time, connected to our ancient past. And if this is so, I thought, is this 'channel 'a two way transport? Do we call upon our ancient ancestors when we tap into ancient memories? When we knead bread, stir soup, breathe in or cook with an exotic spice from

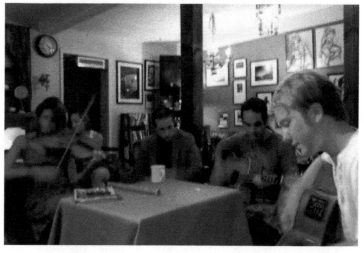

another part of the world? I began to wonder if the spirits of my ancestors were sitting in my kitchen. I felt peaceful and content in the kitchen and had a sense that I was never alone there, even if it appeared that way.

Whether we believe our ancestor spirits are hanging out with us in the kitchen or not, kitchens are still magical places and energetic portals. Why? Because humans are powerful, magical beings. We affect everything we touch and gaze upon. And every ingredient we touch in the kitchen will be eaten by those we love. Every space we occupy is an energetic portal because we are in it, creating thoughts, emotions and intentions. A clean, well-tended kitchen in which food is prepared with care and love will provide families with food that is as nourishing for body and soul as a magical elixir. Kitchens that are not honored, kept clean, tended to and are related to with dread and distain for food preparation will produce food that is as assaultive to the body and the soul as poison.

The food we prepare will always hold our magic. And like temples, our kitchens will always hold the energy and intentions we bring to them. The question is, will we create elixirs or poisons? The choice is ours.

Cooking with Love

I kept a stool next to my prep table because almost every day someone came into the kitchen to sit and share a story or ask for advice. People were drawn to the kitchen like a warm hearth on a cold day. I believe the kitchen is the heart of any home and the heart of any restaurant. I had become aware of the connection between the energy of our

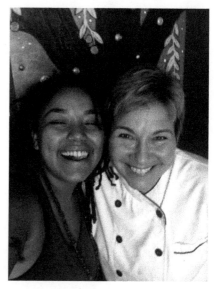

kitchen and the way our customers experienced the food. There was so much love in that kitchen! The young women who worked with me - Bridget, Keahi, and Taylor - were intuitive and empathic. We were all conscious of the energy we brought into the kitchen. I developed the morning ritual of taking a salt bath before coming to work every day, we consciously invited laughter and routinely burnt sage to clear the space.. Even though we held an awareness about the energy in our kitchen and the care with which we prepared the food, I was still surprised by the comments my customers often made about how our food made them feel. These were not fancy dishes artistically plated. I was making soups, breakfast sandwiches, and veggie burgers mostly - yet, people had such strong reactions.

I reflected on my own dining experiences over the years and the times I felt sick after dining out but could not find the cause. While living in New York City for instance, I sometimes had mysterious reactions to food I had eaten in a restaurant. Reactions that had nothing to do with an allergic reaction, or food poisoning . What had caused such negative reactions to a perfectly good dish? As my awareness grew in my own kitchen, I thought more and more about the energy of other kitchens, in fact all kitchens. I thought about food cooked by angry people, whether they are over-worked and under-paid cooks in restaurants or cooks abusing drugs or an angry parent preparing dinner.

I thought about my own childhood. How the arguments my parents had often erupted at the dinner table. How I carried my stress in my stomach and often got stomach aches when upset. Had I always been sensitive to the energy around food? How many people have no idea how affected they are by the negative energy in a kitchen?

As my awareness and curiosity about the effects of kitchen energy grew, I pondered the energetic path to one's stomach. How did the energy from someone preparing food flow to the person eating it? Was it the "ambient energy" of a kitchen that was 'absorbed 'by the food? Maybe. But it occurred to me that we can be directly affected by the energy that flows out of us - from our hands and eyes and the energetic field around us. Just think about the power of eye contact and touch. I became aware of my hands and eyes when preparing food. How could I make sure that the food I was preparing on a daily basis was "made with love"? I became more conscious of my facial expression and thoughts while preparing food. I softened my eyes and kept my heart open. I made a promise to never prepare food while angry or upset.

When I read about Dr. Emoto's experiments with water, the mechanics of what I had been imagining became clear. Cooking with love is a real thing, I thought. And unfortunately, cooking with negative emotions like anger is real too. Dr. Emoto's experiments involved assessing the impact of human intention and emotion on the structure of water. It turns out water is affected on a molecular level by human intentions and emotions. If this concept is applied to food preparation, considering the water content of most food, one can deduce that at the very least, the intentions and emotions of the cooks and food preparers change the molecular structure of the food they are handling.

One day I unknowingly broke my promise to never prepare food while angry or upset. I was going through an upsetting break up at the time and, to make matters worse, it was my birthday. On this particular morning, I arrived still teary eyed from a conversation I had just had and could not shake the sadness. I stood at the griddle making breakfast sandwiches and fighting back tears while Bridget diverted any would-be visitors from the kitchen. It was our

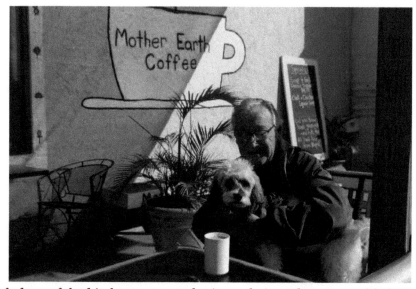

routine to keep the back door of the kitchen open, to let in cool air and so we could chat through the screen with customers who liked to sit under the wonderful old mango tree. On this particular morning, Bri, a regular, quietly ate her egg sandwich on the bench under the mango tree. When she was finished, she stood at the kitchen door and said, "I don't know why I feel so sad, but I do this morning." When I heard this, my mind flashed to the scene from *Like Water For Chocolate* when the young broken-hearted sister cried into the wedding cake she was making and caused the whole wedding party the next day to break into tears shortly after eating it. I ran to the bathroom, splashed cold water on my face and looked into the mirror. "You will not make sad food for your customers." Whether or not my sadness had gotten into Bri's breakfast sandwich made no difference to me. I would not bring sadness ever again into the kitchen.

This promise was challenged two years later when Terry Murphy, a beloved, loyal customer and my mentor chef, passed away. Sadness disturbed my sleep that night and

I woke still weepy. I called my staff and told them I was too sad to work in the kitchen, they would have to cover for me.

I have learned that with awareness comes responsibility. The more we are aware of the ways in which our energy - positive and negative - affects those around us, the more responsibility we must take to make more conscious choices. If we learn that the care and energy with which we prepare food will affect the ones we love on a cellular level, then cooking with love is simply the right thing to do.

The Mango Tree

My little cafe had a 150 year old mango tree outside the kitchen door. The tree get so close to the building that a bough had been cut off to avoid encroaching on the roof. This left a large 'mirror 'section of the tree facing my door, adding even more mystery to its appearance. Not everyone can feel the energy of a tree, but those who can, felt this tree's magnificence. The branches above leaned over the roof of my little place, and the roots ran beneath it. In a way, my little cafe was "hugged" or held by her energetic arms.

Clairvoyants stopped by the cafe and commented on its "energy". What could it be?, we wondered. Then it occurred to me—or perhaps the idea was planted in my consciousness by the spirits there—that the energy of the place had so much to do with the energy of that amazing tree. It had been witness to so much here. Indigenous people had lived here. Some may have buried their dead on the roots of this tree, as was the tradition of so many.

I placed a bench under the tree and began to invite those who were a bit dashed about, heartbroken or sad to have their coffee or tea under her canopy. I called the space under her braces the "intensive care unit'. I even placed weary plants there to soak in her healing atmosphere. People began to report feeling better after spending time with her. Some brought her gifts. Little gem stones, shells and wind chimes.

"There is a spirit who lives in that tree," a woman said one day. "I'd like to come by when you are closed and sit with her. Maybe I can find out more for you." I didn't think anything of it. At the time it seemed like a quirky idea. But the next day, the woman arrived at my cafe, wide-eyed. "I have news for you!" she said. "I talked to the spirit of the tree."

Now here is where folks will either say, " Oh, that's so cool!" or they'll say, "You gotta be kidding me." You may want to stop reading here if you are the latter because it's about to get weirder.

The woman said the tree is occupied by the spirit of an indigenous young woman. A healer. A medicine woman. And that the tree was a kind of temple for her. People had come to her there. She had green eyes, the woman said. Very green eyes. And her name—the name that came to her—was "Jade". I loved the story and began to connect with the energy of the tree, taking a few minutes every day before launching into my work, to sit under the tree and think of her. What began to formulate in my mind was a softer sounding name. The J is an H sound, I kept hearing. The J is an H sound. One day it occurred to me that the correct pronunciation of the green eyed spirit was Hade. Pronounced "Ha-day".

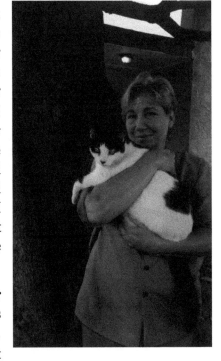

Whether there is a spirit of an indigenous healer in that mango tree or whether the tree itself has its own powerful sentience, that is up to our own beliefs. Most people don't believe animals have sentience, let alone trees and plants. What a world we would inhabit, if it was commonplace to acknowledge that all life on Earth has sentience! What I can tell you is that beautiful tree outside my kitchen door gave us great comfort. She drew people to her and they gathered under her shade. She bore witness to our laughter, our stories, our kisses and tears, just as she had 150 years ago when the people who gathered beneath her told different stories in a tongue that has been lost to this land but not lost to her.

Spirit Daughters

I have had no children of my own, no biological children. There was a moment in my late thirties, as the window was narrowing on this experience, that I attempted unsuccessfully to have a child. This I believe, as with all experiences in my life, was for the best. At the time, I had no idea it was possible to have what I now call "spirit daughters".

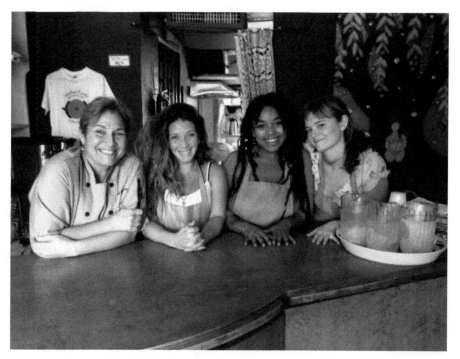

But my cafe was a vortex of manifestation which brought me all manner of experiences. Some heartbreaking, some heart filling, all heart expanding. Among the many souls who entered through the chiming door of my cafe were Bridget and Taylor.

They entered in very different ways, just as children do naturally. Every child has a different birth.

Bridget entered my cafe one afternoon during her high school spring break. She had been looking for jobs in the neighborhood. I was still a one woman operation and had sent away numerous young people who had approached me about working in my "cool" coffeehouse cafe. I was in the middle of preparing some soup in the kitchen when she arrived and had no time to talk to her, but something about her drew me. I asked her to come back the next day when I would have time talk to her. I went about my business in the kitchen and thought about what I could offer her. I had already decided to hire her, but wasn't sure yet for what.

When she arrived the next day we chatted about school, art, coffee and food. She was perfect for Mother Earth. I offered her a job helping with lunch deliveries and the counter. When she arrived for work the following Saturday, she brought a bike specially decorated to deliver lunch for the coffeehouse, with silk flowers and ivy adorning the wicker basket on the front.

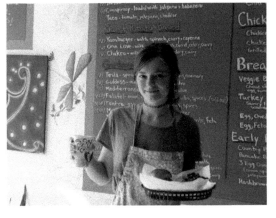

Bridget and I had a morning routine in which we sat with our favorite tea or a cup of coffee under the mango tree and talked about the dreams we had the night before and whatever magical experiences may have occurred since the last time we saw each other. I was always intent on feeding her each shift and she was my taste tester for every new dish or concoction I developed. I remember having a dream once in which Bridget was my daughter. We were cave dwellers and we sat in a dark cave, she lying on her side by the fire, and me sitting next to my male partner. I was upset and fearful because she was not eating. We were cooking meat over the fire and she was refusing to

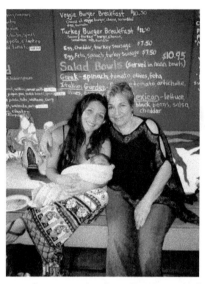

eat it. "This is a denser place," I implored, "We must eat denser food to survive here." I began to cry in my dream. I was distraught because I thought my daughter was going to starve herself to death. I was still crying as I woke. When I shared the dream with Bridget, we both agreed that this ancient history between us had everything to do with my asking her a few times a shift, "Are you hungry? What would you like to eat?" Then carefully preparing a plate for her. Bridget worked at the cafe until we closed the doors for good. Now she comes to visit me from time to time, and I delight in making some of her favorite dishes for her. There is always a feeling of preciousness in these moments, when she shares glimpses of her life. Her art, her music, her lovers, and sometimes her sadness. She plays bass in a band and works in a Miami restaurant. Bridget is my first spirit daughter. Taurus. Earth and stubbornness, musical and epicurean. Sometimes still overwhelmed to tears by the world and its occupants. Tears come easily in the safe space we fold around us, like a cave with a warm fire.

Taylor was born and raised in Lake Worth but did not walk into my cafe until 2014, on the one year anniversary of her mother's death. I remember we hit it off right away. There was a familiarity in our connection. She had her littlest one, Payton, with her. As we chatted, the cafe got busy and soon I had a line at the counter. To this day, Taylor loves telling the story of grabbing an apron from the kitchen and helping me through the lunch rush that day. Regulars came into the cafe and asked, "Who is that behind the counter?"

"Oh, that's Taylor," I responded.

"A new employee?" they asked.

"No," I laughed. "I just met her."

Taylor was a lifesaver that day and I decided to hire her for my busy lunches from that point on. Taylor and I have more of a playful relationship. A different kind of vibe. We both agreed we had been in each other's lives many times before. Taylor put it best when she said, "We've been everything to each other. Parents, children, lovers, friends."

Taylor lives in Tennessee with her four children and husband now. This June, just a few days into my summer vacation, I traveled from my home in South Florida to Tennessee to help prepare her for the home birth of her fourth child. We walked up into the mountains together and stepped over 300 million year old rocks. We sipped tea under majestic trees. I lay quietly outside her room as her contractions came more intensely and as her son gave his first tiny cry in this world. That felt familiar, too. She is my second spirit daughter. Sagittarius. All fire. All heart. Theatrical. Always in motion. "You and I," she says, "We are older than bones." We laugh. Laughter comes easily between us, like an unspoken language that says *We have been here so long, we need little else from each other but laughter.*

Zoey the Cat

A few years after Mother Earth had opened, on a cool autumn evening, just before Open Mic Night, a beautiful tuxedo cat with magnetic green eyes walked through our front door. She was quite nonchalant about it. She hung out by the door and greeted people as they came in.

"Is this your cat?" they'd asked.

"No," I'd reply. "She just wandered in."

"She's beautiful!"

"Why not keep her?"

I put food out for her and she began to come around every day. I discovered she was sleeping by the front door at night, or under the mango tree outside my kitchen door. People reported seeing her curled up outside the cafe all hours of the night.

"You should keep her," they said. "It looks like she wants to stay."

After a few weeks, people began to ask her name. I decided I should name her so I called her Zoey. Soon, everyone who came to Mother Earth knew our cafe cat named Zoey.

For her part, Zoey seemed to love her new home. I knew I was breaking food establishment rules by letting her hang out inside, but my customers loved her so much and so did I. Soon, customers were asking for Zoey before they ordered their food!

It turned out, Zoey patrolled the neighborhood at night. She walked a particular parameter. Often, customers reported seeing her on the next street over, leisurely walking along the sidewalk. One day a regular customer, Jesse, came into the cafe with a particularly funny Zoey story. He had been at the bar across the street one night when

Zoey walked in and climbed up on the bar stool next to him. The bartender was going to shoo her away when Jesse told him he knew her.

"She just sat there like she was one of us shooting the shit," Jesse said.

For years Zoey hung out at Mother Earth, greeting customers, napping on the cool tile floor, keeping out the mice, and being a friend to anyone who needed a furry headbutt to remind them that everything was going to be alright.

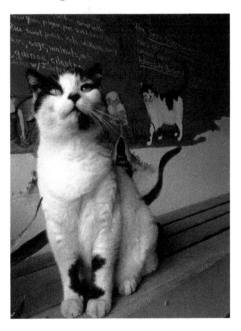

When Bridget created the whimsical artwork around our wall menu, Zoey's image mingled with gnomes, fairies and dragonflies under mushroom houses. She was as magical.

When it came time for the cafe to close, many customers were concerned about Zoey.

"You should take her with you," they said.

But Zoey was and will always be a free spirit. She was not a house cat and would not surrender to the domesticated life. I learned that she was wildly popular in the neighborhood. She made "stops" at many homes—where she was lovingly fed and cooed. And I learned she went by many names. Zoey had just been the name we knew her by at Mother Earth.

So, Zoey, like the rest of us, moved on from the cafe. I imagine she wanders by, from time to time, just like her human friends from those cafe days, and she may pause as we do when we drive by, and remember the love, the laughter, the food, and those precious furry headbutts.

Gene, the Angel

I believe that when one is about to enter a period of great challenge, there are warning signs. Kind of like the universe putting up signs that say "Bump Ahead", or more accurately, "Cliff Ahead". Our attachment to the way things are usually prevents us from seeing the signs at all or perhaps giving them more assuring interpretations. But then, sometimes there are angels or messengers that cross our path right at the most important moments. Gene was that for me.

Gene was a little man who came to my cafe regularly. He was short and stout and brown skinned with curly grey hair and round wire rimmed glasses. I was usually in the kitchen when he came for his soup and tea or a muffin and coffee. Bridget would usually wait on him. On this one particular day in mid-September of 2016, Gene came into the cafe and ordered a muffin and coffee and sat at the table closest to the kitchen door. For some reason I had to go out to the counter to get something and Gene beckoned me as soon as he saw me.

"Hi Patti, " He said, "I have a question about your muffins."

I could have stood at the counter and answered his question but for some reason on this particular day, I went over to his table and sat across from him. He had such a pleasant demeanor, his round face in a continuous smile, his brown eyes sparkling behind the round lenses of his glasses. Gene wore a crisp white shirt and dress trousers, but carried a backpack. I remember thinking that was an odd combination.

"I was going to ask you about the salt content in your muffins," he began.

"Very low, Gene." I said. "And I only use Himalayan pink salt."

"Yes, very nice." Gene continued. "I always enjoy the energy of your place. I feel nourished, body and spirit. You have created quite a special place here."

I smiled and began telling him about the magnificent tree outside my kitchen door whose roots run underneath, but he gently interrupted me, as if he didn't really notice that I was about to tell him a story.

"You have always had such a wonderful imagination," he said, his eyes looking now into some distant place. "You have always been so creative."

I stopped talking and listened. Perhaps I held my breath. Those seemed strange comments to make by a man who did not know me. Then he continued.

"I remember watching you as a child," he continued. My heart dropped. Was Gene crazy? Creepy? "You had such an imagination then. You were always creating new things." He was smiling at something distant, as if rewinding a tape. He spoke slowly, pausing for a few moments between sentences. "Life was not easy for you, but you never let your heart become bitter. You never lost hope. This is a precious quality."

A single tear escaped my eye and traveled slowly down my cheek.

"I can't lose hope." I whispered. I didn't think Gene was crazy anymore. I believed he was a messenger of some kind. He continued talking, his smile never leaving his face. He talked as if he had followed me throughout my life. How could this be? Who was he?

"You have come into my cafe many times but we never sat and talked like this..."

"It was time." Gene said.

"Why?"

"You are about to go through a transition." Gene said. He was gathering his backpack and pushing in his chair. I didn't want him to leave. I stood up and he put his hands on my shoulders.

"You are adorable," he said looking deeply into my eyes. "Remember that". I wondered what that meant because he didn't say it like most people do. Like a compliment about how one looks. It was more like 'having the quality of being adored'.

He hugged me and was gone.

I stepped into the kitchen, still teary eyed and said to Bridget, "Bridget you won't believe the conversation I just had with Gene. It was like he knew me my whole life!"

Bridget smiled and said, "I've always thought Gene was a little angel."

I never saw Gene again.

One week later, Hurricane Matthew was bearing down on the east coast of Florida. I thought to myself, *Is this the transition Gene was referring to?* Would this hurricane destroy my little cafe? We all hunkered down, boarding windows and doors, and waited for the storm to pass. Hurricane Matthew was not as destructive as we had feared and I was back in business the very next day.

Two weeks later, however, I would learn that my cafe would have to close when my lease was up in November. The new owners of our building did not want a full kitchen on the premises. Just as I was getting ready for a record season, we would have to close. I had six weeks to clear the space. I also lived in the apartment above my cafe. The leases for both were up at the same time. I decided to leave my apartment too because I could not bear the thought of living above the space that once was my beloved little cafe. In six short weeks I was without a livelihood and a home. Gene's words began to feel like an understatement.

Now, on the five year anniversary of the closing of my cafe, *Wildflowers and Wooden Spoons*, my second book in the *Wildflower* series is being released and with it, the recipes and stories of an unforgettable ten-year experience. Gene was right. I was about to experience a transition from one life to another. I've lived multiple lives in this lifetime, often marked by transitions from one geographical place to another. This journey was not marked by a change of place so much as more mysterious changes brought by an inward journey of self-discovery. Sometimes we experience these great changes during the period of our lives marked by the 'Saturn Return', every twenty-eight years. Sometimes these great changes are represented by a flurry of outward changes, and sometimes the journey is inward, a sort of Dark Night of the Soul. Life transitions are inevitable. Necessary. And there are always signs if we choose to pay attention. Sometimes, if we are lucky, we may get a visit from a gentle angel like Gene who reminds us that we are adored by countless unseen ancestors and an ever watchful Creator.

Now, Reflecting Back

I am completing this cookbook in the summer of 2021, four years after the close of Mother Earth Sanctuary Cafe. I've had time to take in the lessons and the treasures of the experience of owning and operating such a gathering place in the community. Even the concept of "gathering places" feels almost nostalgic in 2021, but humans are meant to gather and we will find ways to create gathering places again.

I didn't know what I was doing, really, as a business owner. I was building the bridge as I crossed the river and, to extend that metaphor a bit more, I often found myself dangling precariously over the raging waters of defeat. I was, as they say "undercapitalized", like so many small business owners who create a business on a dream and the desire to serve. I had originally opened a coffeehouse with my partner at the time, but four months in, our relationship dissolved and I found myself a 'one woman operation'. I had already left the security of a teaching job and now found myself barely able to keep a roof over my head. What got me through those first two years of mostly dangling from my poorly strung-together bridge was my own

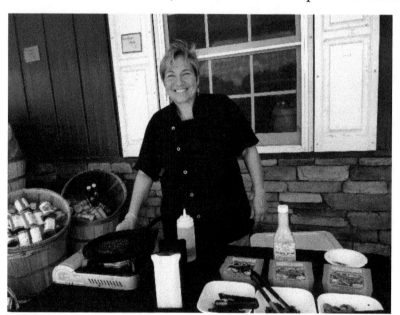

stubbornness and the generosity of so many people in the Lake Worth community. Laura, Jackie and Steph offered me places to stay. Jen worked for tips on Open Mic Nights and brought me home cooked meals. Bryce did milk runs. Cleo helped out during the day and offered moral support. Local artists brought art to hang on the walls. Local

musicians spread the word about Open Mic Nights and established my little 850 square foot place as "the place to be on Thursday nights".

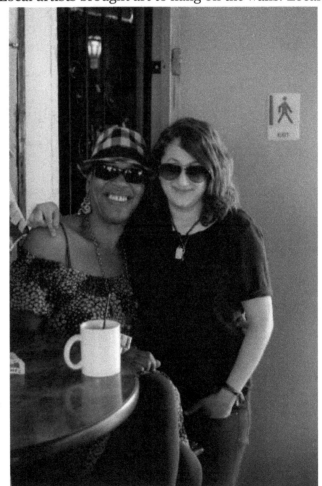

The little place took on a life of its own and anchored a certain magic. People fell in love there. (I certainly did). People met soul mates and friends. They wrote poetry and affirmations in my coffee table journals. They came to share their new girlfriends and they came when they were heartbroken. They came to say good-bye when college or a new job called them away, and reconnected with family and friends on the comfy couches when they returned. I watched teenagers grow up and others grow old. I watched the steady decline of two beloved regulars and grieved their loss. The morning "Miss Cleo" (who had been a regular for years) died, Channel 12 news showed up at my cafe. The cafe had been her safe place, too, and the only address the local news could find that was associated with the reclusive Miss Cleo.

I had thought my cafe would go on indefinitely. I had no Plan B. Silly me. But sometimes when we get swept up in our dreams, we just don't want to think of their possible end. In the fall of 2016, I was informed by the new owners of the building that they did not want a full restaurant on the premises. I had six weeks until the end of my lease. Six weeks to close out a ten year experience and weigh my options for the future. It was exactly the transition "Gene the Angel" had referenced and I was not prepared.

In the years that have passed since then, I have had the opportunity to focus inward, focus on my own growth. Though there are many people who have asked me to open another cafe, I will not step into that experience again. The year 2021 and the lockdowns have shown us how fragile those businesses are. The profit margins are so narrow, it has been impossible for the majority of independent food outlets to survive. Instead, I have focused on teaching and writing. *Wildflowers and Wooden Spoons* is the second of three in my *Wildflowers* series. I have two more books slated for 2022 and a series of novellas after that. I host a podcast and enjoy being a guest on other podcasts. I think we live in interesting times, even with the extreme challenges. I plan on spending the next 20 years making a contribution to the whole, to new and emerging paradigms in thinking, business, spirituality and collaboration. Perhaps it is not a time for any of us to be anchored to one tiny location but to be moving about, connecting, exploring and expanding into new realities.

If you were a customer at Mother Earth Sanctuary Cafe, I thank you for being part of my journey and for allowing me to be a part of yours. I hope to share a tea and conversation with you again one day, perhaps in a place neither of us has ever been before. I look forward to that!

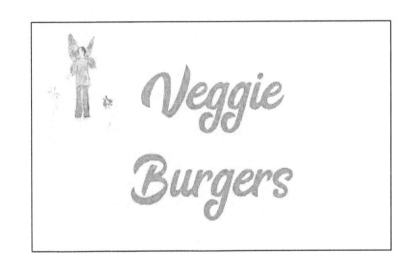

Old School Veggie Burgers

It seems like a funny term to use, "old school" veggie burgers. Veggie burgers haven't been around for that long, have they? The first known commercial veggie burgers were the Boca Burger. For many years—even decades—if one wanted a veggie burger, that was the only choice.

Early in my cafe days, I was expanding the menu and one of my customers, a high school student, requested that I try making veggie burgers because everywhere he went the veggie burgers were terrible. I was certainly up for the challenge and a few weeks later had created my first veggie burger, The Yamburger.

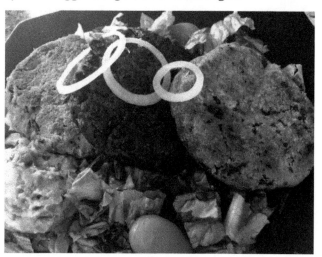

The biggest challenge in creating veggie burgers is how to 'hold them together'. Some commercial veggie burgers contain egg as a binder, many (too many) use soy and others use bulgur wheat. I didn't like any of these options so I experimented with several options for binding my burgers. The best option I discovered was oats. This came to me after considering what a bowl of oatmeal looks like if left out too long. I could also acquire gluten free oats which was exciting because I wanted to produce gluten free veggie burgers. I personally feel much better when I am avoiding gluten in my diet.

There are many perspectives on the gluten question, and much heated debate. I'm not going to get into them here. I try to keep things as simple as possible and free from food ideologies (yep, it's a thing). My perspective on gluten is the same as my perspective on any other food. Listen to your body. If gluten or any other food makes your body uncomfortable, then it's not the right nutrition for your body. I don't get involved in the gluten debate. I just have a private conversation with my own body and make my food decisions accordingly. (For more about my personal journey to a better relationship with my body and to optimal health, check out my book *This Amazing Body*.)

Once I had the challenge of how to bind the burgers solved, I could create burgers from a wide range of bases, and that is exactly what I did. I experimented with yams, black beans, garbanzo beans, lentils, quinoa, apple, brown rice, and Jamaican yellow yam. In the end I had created over twenty original veggie burgers, each with their own unique base, herb combination and spices.

The creation of veggie burgers became an art form, beginning with a concept then expanding and enhancing that concept with ingredients. For instance, when I created the Tesla burger (named for the man not the car—this was before the car.), I thought of Nicola Tesla and his legacy. I pondered the concept of free energy. Energy for the body. Protein. Garbanzo beans have more protein than any other bean so I knew the Tesla burger had to be garbanzo based. But what other ingredients would complement this theme? Let's add even more protein, I thought. Pumpkin seeds. Very high in protein. So ground pumpkin seeds were added. Iron is also important for energy. I added spinach. And for some crazy reason, I thought raisins would be a nice compliment. Iron and sweetness. Tesla was a gentle, brilliant and sweet man. A man, unfortunately, too ahead of his time, as out of place in conventional society as raisins in a burger. I pondered what herb would best be suited for such an unusual mix of ingredients. I chose rosemary. "Rosemary," Ophelia had said in Shakespeare's *Hamlet*, "is for remembrance". Rosemary seemed like the best fit for a burger made in Tesla's honor. Now that we have come to appreciate the man, let us remember him with fondness and gratitude. (And by the way, Elon, your car would be more suited for its name if it ran on the kind of electricity Tesla actually studied. Here's hoping you may do that one day.)

When sampling my veggie burgers at Farmer's Markets I was often asked, "Which of your burgers tastes most like meat?" To which I replied, "None of them do. I did not design them to taste like meat." Don't get me wrong. I'm not anti-meat. I think if you want the taste and enjoyment of meat, eat meat. If you want a plant based life, celebrate the plants. I always thought it odd that vegan restaurants offered dishes that emulated meat dishes when there are so many ways to make vegetable based dishes taste uniquely delicious. I think other cultures around the world have done a better job in this way of eating because they use a much wider variety of herbs and spices. Indian food is a wonderful example of this. Even cultures that are not as plant based as Indian culture are able to create satisfying dishes without meat using wonderful spice combinations. In Ethiopian culture, berbere, a common spice combination is used in most dishes, with and without meat.

So, the veggie burgers I created at my cafe and the recipes contained in this cookbook are not veggie burgers that taste like meat. There are plenty of options now for people who are looking for that experience. The Beyond Burger and the Impossible Burger have hit the market and skyrocketed in popularity. Restaurants wanting to offer vegan selections will offer these on their menu. But, just like so much of the processed vegan food sold in supermarkets, the problem with these burgers is that they are highly processed and a far from whole food goodness. If you want to live a plant based life for whatever reasons you have chosen, it is important not to sacrifice your health in the process.

The best solution is to get in the kitchen as often as possible and make your own. Want veggie burgers? Make your own! It's not that hard and once you get started you may find, as I did, that the creative process takes over and you will have a freezer full of whole food, handmade veggie burgers named after your favorite world figures. Think of it. What would a Gandhi burger taste like? A Barbara Streisand burger? Why not create a burger that helps you recall that favorite vacation? The possibilities are endless. And honestly, any food you create with joy and love in your own kitchen will bring joy and love to you on a cellular level. Bet you didn't think making your own veggie burgers could get that deep, did you?

Black Bean Burger

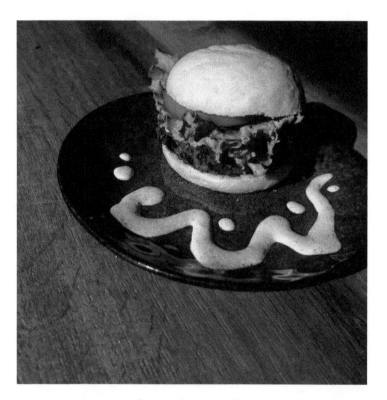

Black beans are very versatile and so is this burger. Here is the recipe for the basic Black Bean burger and from this base you can create endless variations, just as I did at my cafe. If you like your burgers with heat, you can add jalapeños. If you like cheese, you can mix in shredded cheddar or a Mexican cheese mix. Like tomato? Add some diced tomato. You get the picture. This is how I was able to create so many variations of veggie burgers at my cafe. I simply started with a base—black bean, garbanzo, lentil, sweet potato—then took it in different directions. You can be as creative as you want to be with veggie burgers, and while you're at it, have fun naming your creations. This simple creative process helps bring joy into the kitchen. And a joyful kitchen makes joyful food.

Ingredients

2 cans organic black beans, rinsed, drained

1 cup quinoa, cooked, cooled

1 sweet onion, chopped

3 cloves garlic, minced

1/2 cup fresh cilantro, de-stemmed, chopped

1 teaspoon chili powder

1 teaspoon ground cumin

1 teaspoon Himalayan Pink salt, or sea salt

1/2 teaspoon pepper

1/2 cups oats, ground

Directions

1. Put one can of black beans aside. Mash 1 can of black beans (a blender works best).

2. Put the mashed black beans in a mixing bowl.

3. Add quinoa, onion, garlic, cilantro and spices and mix well.

4. Add whole black beans and mix.

5. At this point, it's good to taste the dough and make sure it is salted enough for your taste.

6. Add the ground oats and mix well.

7. Form patties.

8. Put your choice of oil in a pan or griddle. Set on medium high.

9. Place burgers in pan. Cook until browned (4 - 5 minutes) then flip.

10. Add cheese (optional) to melt.

11. Serve on a roll or greens.

12. Extra patties can be frozen.

Variations

I had two other popular black bean based burgers on my menu. Here are their directions.

Aztec Burger

Use the Black Bean Burger base. Add additional 1 teaspoon of chili spice, 1/2 teaspoon cumin, 2 fresh chopped jalapeño peppers, 1 fresh tomato, diced, 1/4 cup fresh corn off the cob (optional).

Conspiracy Burger

This burger is for 'heat 'lovers! Use the Black Bean Burger base and add 1/2 teaspoon cayenne pepper and 4 chopped fresh jalapeño peppers.

The Yamburger

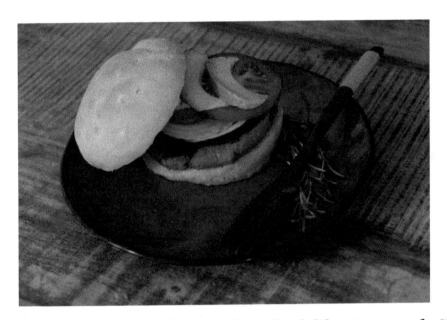

My early menu was mostly comfort food like Mac and Cheese, Shepherd's Pie, and Collard Greens with Smoked Turkey Wings. One day a young customer approached me with a request. He asked if I would try making a veggie burger because everywhere he went, the veggie burgers were terrible. This intrigued me, and loving a good foodie challenge, I set to work.

In no time, I learned that the world of veggie burgers in 2009 was a sad one, with limited choices, and those choices were loaded with salt and soy.

I decided to create a veggie burger with no egg, soy, dairy or gluten. One afternoon, while preparing a lunch special, I took a closer look at the bowl of mashed sweet potato. What a pretty and nutritious base for a burger, I thought. So I set about creating my first veggie burger, The Yamburger. I loved curry with yam so this became the predominant spice. For color, I added spinach and dark red kidney beans. What a pretty burger! The challenge, as always, is finding a way to 'keep it together'. I used a combination of oats and garbanzo beans. When I offered samples to customers and got enthusiastic thumbs up, I decided to keep creating veggie burgers. Within five years my little cafe became known as a veggie burger cafe with as many as twenty veggie burgers on the menu.

It all began with a simple request and the creation of my very first veggie burger, The Yamburger!

Ingredients

4 cups mashed baked yams (5-6 baked sweet potatoes)

1 cup chopped fresh spinach

1 cup dark red kidney beans, rinsed

3/4 cups chopped onion

1/4 cup garlic, minced

1 cup cooked quinoa

1 tablespoon curry powder

1 teaspoon cumin powder

1/2 teaspoon cayenne

1 teaspoon sea salt

1/2 teaspoon pepper

1 cup ground oats (gluten-free oats recommended)

Directions

1. Put mashed sweet potatoes in a large bowl.

2. Add spinach, kidney beans, onion, garlic, quinoa and all spices.

3. Mix well, preferably with your hands.

4. Slowly add the ground oats and mix with hands.

5. Form patties and set them aside.

6. Heat a non-stick or cast iron pan to medium-high heat.

7. Add your choice of oil to the pan.

8. Add the patties to the pan and let cook until slightly brown (About 4 - 5 minutes) on one side.

9. Flip the burger and let it cook until browned on the other side.

10. Serve on your choice of bread. Add lettuce and tomato, if you like.

11. If you are a cheese lover, I recommend either feta or goat cheese on this burger.

12. Add your choice of cheese while cooking to melt or as you serve.

13. This burger is also wonderful when served in a wrap with micro greens.

Variations:

I had two other sweet potato based burgers that were quite popular. Here are their directions.

Chakra burger

Use the Yamburger base without the red kidney beans and spinach. Add I cup kale, 1/2 cup celery, and 1 cup mashed eggplant (peel, cut into thick slices, bake, then mash)

One Love Burger

Use the Yamburger base without the red kidney beans and spinach. Add 1 cup pigeon peas, 1/2 cup fresh chopped carrot, and 1/2 cup chopped fresh celery, and an additional teaspoon of curry.

Dragon Burger

At the time I created the Dragon Burger, I was, I'll admit, on a bit of an 'elementals' kick. Fairies, dragons, unicorns. I wanted to create burgers that honored each mythical being with carefully selected ingredients, herbs and spices. So when I decided to create the Dragon Burger, I pondered the most appropriate base. Not beans. No, no, no. Not sweet potato or potato, either. No squash would do. This base had to be earthy, firm and strong. It had to have a presence! When I began to work with Jamaican yellow yam, I knew I had found the perfect base for a Dragon Burger.

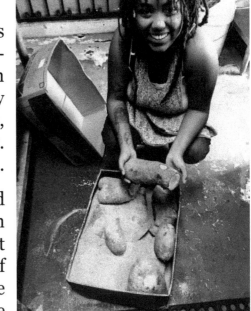

The Jamaican yellow yam is intimidating. Covered in a thick bark-like skin, you have to approach it with respect (and a very sharp and heavy knife). And unlike other yams, Jamaican yellow yam is not sweet. Again, most appropriate for a Dragon.

Next, I contemplated the herbs and spices. I wanted to accentuate both earth and fire with every ingredient because that's what dragons are—of deep earth, dwelling in caves and the interior of mountains, and intense fire. I chose pigeon peas for their beautiful brown-green color and texture, reminding me a dragon's scales, sage for its earthiness and wisdom (dragons are old and their wisdom is beyond our comprehension), carrot for its rooted earthy sweetness, fire color and texture, smoked paprika for its wonderful deep red color and aroma (like a sleeping dragon), cayenne for fire, scotch bonnet peppers for more fire!

Ingredients

8 cups Jamaican yellow yam, cooked, mashed

16 ounces pigeon peas

1 bunch fresh sage, de-stemmed, chopped

1 cup fresh carrot, peeled and roughly chopped

1 cup fresh onion, chopped

5 cloves garlic, minced

4 tablespoons smoked paprika

1 tablespoon cayenne

5 fresh Scotch bonnet peppers, seeded, chopped finely

1/2 cup ground oats

2 teaspoons Himalayan Pink salt

1 cup coconut milk

Directions

1. To prepare the Jamaican yellow yam, peel, cut up and place in boiling water. Boil until soft enough to pierce with a fork (20 - 25 minutes), drain and set aside to cool. Place in a bowl with 1/2 cup of coconut milk and mash until smooth, using the remainder of the coconut milk if needed. The consistency should be like

thick, stiff, lumpy mashed potatoes. If you want your yam base to be completely smooth, use a food processor for mixing and process a little at a time.

2. Place your yam mix in a large bowl and add the pigeon peas, sage, carrot, onion, garlic and mix. Putting on gloves and mixing with your hands is best. Once it is thoroughly blended add the remainder of the ingredients except for the ground oats. Mix well by hand. The ground oats is the binder so add it slowly and mix in.

3. Once your mixture is done, form patties. The suggested size is 6 ounces, but you can make a variety of sizes including sliders. If you have more patties than you need, you can put the extra in the fridge (they will be good for up to four days), or freezer. These burgers freeze well.

4. Set your non-stick cooking surface or cast iron pan to medium high heat. Use oil, butter or pan spray to keep the burgers from sticking. Cook until browned to your liking on one side, then flip the burger and cook until browned on the other side. Usually 5 - 6 minutes per side. If you like cheese on your burgers, we found that goat cheese worked well on this burger but I recommend the cheese you like best. Serve on a bun or cut up on a salad. Any of my burger sauce recipes will work with this burger.

Coexist Burger

The Coexist Burger was the last veggie burger I created at my cafe. I wanted to create a veggie burger with a variety of beans and often joked that, "If these beans can coexist, so can human beans." I used black beans, red beans and white beans with a good deal of mushrooms for umami, and rounded out these ingredients with herbes de Provence, a nod to the French who had always welcomed our intellectuals, musicians and artists of color. People like James Baldwin, Richard Wright, Josephine Baker and Nina Simone. The Coexist Burger was the most labor intensive and complex of my burger creations. "This is fitting," I remember thinking, "coexistence takes time." True coexistence, the kind that evolves naturally—not by legislation—is a dance that begins with the dancers across the room, moving in closer circles until they touch, hold and spin together. A dance of exploration and discovery that leads us home to the beginning—to Eden, perhaps—where the beauty and breathtaking diversity of our human family blooms and grows.

Ingredients

1 can organic black beans

1 can organic red beans

1 can organic Northern white beans

1 cup sliced mushrooms

4 stalks celery, chopped

2 carrots, peeled, well chopped

1 large sweet onion, chopped

4 cloves fresh garlic, minced

2 cups cooked quinoa

2 tablespoons Herbes de Provence

1 teaspoon Himalayan Pink salt

1/2 teaspoon pepper

1/2 cup ground oats

Directions

1. Place a large, well-oiled skillet over medium high heat and add onion and garlic. Sauté until the onion is translucent. Add mushroom, carrot, celery, Herbes de Provence, 1 teaspoon of salt and 1/2 teaspoon of pepper. Sauté until carrot and celery are soft, then take off heat. Drain liquid from mixture and set aside to cool.

2. Drain and rinse each can of beans, then put half of each in a bowl and set aside, and the other half in a large mixing bowl and mash. Add the cooked quinoa to the mashed beans and mix. Add the cooked vegetable and mushrooms and mix well. Fold in the whole beans. Add the ground oats and mix well by hand. Form patties.

3. To cook patties, place a well-oiled skillet over medium high heat. Place patties in skillet and cook until slightly browned on one side, about 5 minutes. Flip pattie and cook until slightly browned, another 3 - 5 minutes.

4. Serve warm on a roll or wrap or over salad.

Tesla Burger

Let me say firstly that this burger was not named after a car. It predates the Musk invention. I created the Tesla Burger as a homage to the man, Nicola Tesla, the father of free energy. Every ingredient was chosen with this intention. Garbanzo beans, for instance, have more protein than any other bean. Energy! Pumpkin seeds have more protein than other seeds. Energy! You get the picture. Iron is represented by spinach and raisins. Rosemary for remembrance. Let us remember the man and his great work, which is not fairly represented by cars that run on electricity generated by generators. The electricity Tesla was harnessing comes from our atmosphere and is free. Just saying.

Ingredients

2 cans organic garbanzo beans, rinsed, drained

1 cup quinoa, cooked, cooled

1/2 cup chopped fresh spinach

1/2 cup ground pumpkin seeds

1/2 cup raisins

2 fresh limes (juiced)

1/2 sweet onion, chopped

3 cloves garlic, minced

1/4 cup fresh rosemary, chopped fine

1 teaspoon Himalayan Pink salt or sea salt

1/2 teaspoon pepper

1 cup ground oats (gluten-free oats recommended)

Cooking oil of choice

Directions

1. Using a food processor, process the garbanzo beans until smooth and place in a mixing bowl.

2. Add quinoa, spinach, ground pumpkin seed, raisins, onion, garlic, rosemary, lime juice, salt and pepper. Mix thoroughly by hand. Slowly mix in the ground oats.

3. Form into patties.

4. Cover the bottom of a frying pan or cast iron skillet or griddle with oil and set on medium high heat.

5. Place patties in the pan and cook until lightly browned on one side (about 3-4 minutes), then flip and brown the other side. If cheese is desired, put on the browned side to melt. (Recommended cheeses for the Tesla burger are feta and goat.)

6. Serve on a roll or over salad.

Falafel Burger

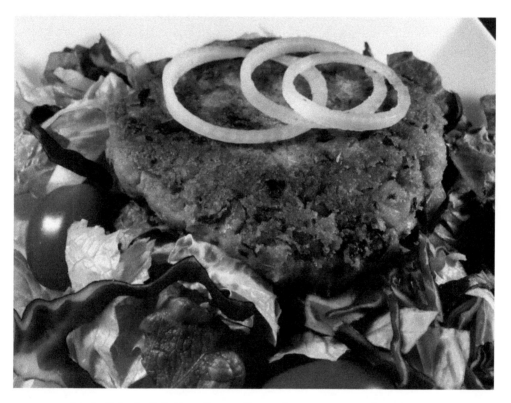

Mmmmm. Falafel. I think of my days in New York City when I smell fresh falafel. Falafel represents peace to me. It is a favorite food from the Middle East across all borders. It was this intention—peace—with which I made my first batch of Falafel Burgers. I sometimes wonder if food prepared and served with such intentions in great enough numbers might contribute significantly to world peace.

Ingredients

2 cans organic garbanzo beans, rinsed, drained

1 cup fresh cilantro, de-stemmed, chopped

1 cup fresh parsley, de-stemmed, chopped

1/2 cup tahini

1 onion, chopped

3 cloves garlic, minced

3 limes (juiced)

1 tablespoon ground cumin

3/4 cups oats, ground

1 teaspoon Himalayan Pink salt or sea salt

1/2 teaspoon pepper

Directions

1. Process garbanzo beans in blender or food processor until smooth. Place in mixing bowl.

2. Add cilantro, parsley, onion, garlic, tahini, lime juice, cumin, salt and pepper. Mix well by hand. Slowly mix in ground oats. Form patties.

3. Put oil of choice in pan and set heat to medium high.

4. Place patties in pan and cook until slightly browned on one side. Flip.

5. Cook until slightly browned on other side. If you like cheese, feta or goat cheese are great compliments to this burger. Once flipped, place cheese choice on browned side to melt. Serve on a roll, wrap or salad.

6. Freeze extra patties.

Turkey Burger

What I hear most from people who do not care for turkey burgers is that they tend to be dry or they just don't have as much flavor. Fair enough. But those problems are easy fixes and if you are looking to reduce your fat intake, turkey burgers are a nice substitute for regular beef burgers.

If you are on a budget (and who isn't these days?) I suggest buying ground turkey in bulk, making a stack of turkey burgers and freezing them. This approach is great for convenience, too!

Ingredients

5 pounds ground turkey (full fat is best)

1 medium onion, chopped fine

4 fresh garlic cloves, minced

1/2 cup fresh sage leaves, chopped fine

1/4 cup oil of choice (olive, grape seed, avocado)

2 tablespoons Worcestershire sauce

1 teaspoon Himalayan Pink salt or sea salt

1/2 teaspoon pepper

Directions

1. Place all ingredients in a large mixing bowl and mix thoroughly with gloved hands. Form into patties sized to your liking. The burger will shrink a bit on the griddle. I like making hearty 8-ounce patties. Place the patties on a tray, cover

and place in the fridge for 30 minutes before cooking. This recipe also makes great turkey meatballs. Any extra burger patties or meatballs can be frozen for future enjoyment.

2. Set griddle or oiled pan on medium high heat and place burgers leaving room between for flipping. Cook 5 - 7 minutes on each side or until cooked to safe internal temperature of 160 degrees. Remove from pan and let set for 3 - 5 minutes. Place on bun with choice of toppings - try my recipe for burger buns and condiments.

Notes

Soups

Soup: Memory, Healing and Connection

Soup is among the oldest foods known to humans all over the world, making it one of our oldest collective memories. The bones from the hunt made primitive soups shared by a whole community. For centuries, kettles over hearths provided a continuous source of sustenance and a way to extract every bit of nourishment from bones, organs, vegetable scraps and roots.

We associate soup with warmth, healing and love. The love of a mother, the love of a healer, the love of Earth herself. Medicine men and women made soups with special ingredients for healing. Soup recipes were handed down through hundreds of generations. Our connection to soup is as strong and deep as our DNA.

If it is true that our DNA holds the memory of our lineages as well as the memory of the human species, soup may be a common memory associated with the very best of human emotions: love, compassion, connection and contentment. It is no wonder we have such warm associations with soup.

When I began to expand my menu from simple coffeehouse selections to a daily cafe menu, I spent some time researching a variety of soups from around the world including the ancient healing Brazilian Yucca Stew, Indian Dahl, and Ethiopian Red Lentil Stew. Many soup recipes used today have been around for centuries and contain the same herbs and spices. If you have ever tasted a food with a spice you have never had before and it mysteriously feels familiar, how is that explained? Or perhaps we crave foods from a particular region of the world which contain certain spices. What is behind such cravings? Is it simply a physical need for certain nutrients? Hardly. I like to consider the possibility that these unexplainable desires for certain foods and spices may be connected to DNA memory of those regions, either through a bloodline or lifetimes.

So the next time you sip soup and tear a piece of bread to go with it, allow yourself a moment to close your eyes and reflect. Imagine all the times your ancient hands may have stirred a pot, held a bowl, and broke off a piece of bread to soak up the last bit of soup. How much better our soup may taste if we allow ourselves to savor the ancient memories of the soups that nourished us so long ago.

Brussels Sprout Bisque

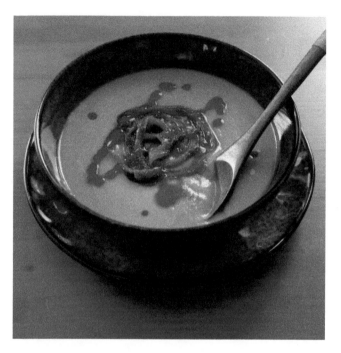

Brussels Sprout Bisque is another simple soup that is so delicious! You may be wondering what raspberry sauce has to do with this soup and why in the world would one put these two together. Some foods are natural compliments like sage and poultry. Some are what I like to call 'secret lovers'. Raspberries and Brussels sprouts are completely unexpected in this way, and, complimented with caramelized onion this bisque becomes a bowl of mischievous delight, served best with a wink.

Ingredients

For the Bisque

2 pounds of fresh Brussels sprouts, washed and cut in half

2 medium onions, chopped

7 cloves fresh garlic, minced

Olive oil

Himalayan pink salt

Pepper

For the Raspberry sauce

1 pack of fresh raspberries, washed

1 lime

1/4 cup regular sugar or monk fruit sweetener or honey (your choice)

For the Caramelized Onion

3 sweet onions, sliced thin

2 tablespoons olive oil

2 tablespoons butter

2 tablespoons sugar or monk fruit sweetener

Himalayan pink salt

Directions

1. Pour 2 tablespoons olive oil in the bottom of a soup pot and put over medium heat. Add onion and garlic and sauté until the onion is translucent. Add a pinch of salt and pepper.

2. Place the Brussels sprouts in the pot and add just enough water to cover them. Cover and let cook until the Brussels sprouts are soft enough to poke through with a fork. (About 20 minutes) Take off the stove and set aside, covered.

3. Add 2 tablespoons of olive oil and 2 tablespoons of butter to a large skillet and place over medium heat. Put the onion in the pan with a pinch of salt and sauté until soft, stirring regularly. Stir in sugar or sweetener, cover, lower heat to medium low and let cook another 10 minutes. off stove and set aside.

4. Add raspberries to a blender. Add the juice of one lime. Add the sugar or sweetener. Blend for 30 seconds. Pour raspberry sauce through a sieve or cheese cloth to remove the seeds. Set seedless sauce aside.

5. Pour the cooked Brussels sprouts and stock into a clean blender. Puree and pour into a soup pot. You may need to do this a few times until all the Brussels sprouts with stock have been pureed and added to the soup pot. Put the pureed Brussels sprouts over medium low heat until sufficiently warmed for serving.

6. Pour into a bowl or crock, top with a generous portion of caramelized onion, drizzle raspberry sauce on top, and serve!

Yucca Stew

When I first expanded the menu at my coffeehouse, I thought soup was a wonderful addition but because my coffeehouse was located in Florida, I thought I could only serve hot soup in the cooler months. I was wrong. My customers liked hot soup all year round. And what a relief! I honestly never warmed to the idea of cold soups.

(Sorry, Gazpacho!)

One of my customers' favorites was a creamy yucca soup. The inspiration for this soup came from a wonderful book called *"Sacred Cookbook"* by Nick Polizzi. The cookbook was a collection of healing recipes from around the world. This particular inspiration comes from Brazil. I made a vegan version of this soup but if you like seafood, shrimp and scallops are a wonderful addition.

Ingredients

3 cups mashed yucca

1/2 t Himalayan Pink salt or sea salt

1 15-ounce can coconut milk

1 cup collard greens, de-stemmed and chopped

1 pound raw shrimp, peeled and deveined

1 pound scallops, thawed

1 cup fresh cilantro, de-stemmed, roughly chopped

1 medium onion, chopped

4 cloves garlic, minced

1 red bell pepper, chopped

2 jalapeño peppers, chopped

3 fresh tomatoes, diced

2 tablespoons coconut oil

Juice of 2 limes

Directions

1. To cook the yucca: Peel and cut up the yucca, removing the hard vein that runs down the middle of the root. Oil a pot 3/4 of the way with water and bring to a boil. Add 1 teaspoon of coconut oil, a pinch of salt, yucca and collard greens. Cook until the yucca is soft enough to pierce with a fork. About 30 minutes.

2. Drain and let cool in a large bowl. Mash with a potato masher until chunks are very small. Remove any stringy pieces or yucca vein you may see. Add the coconut milk and puree with an emersion blender or in a food processor. Return to the pot and set aside.

3. In a large sauté pan, add the coconut oil and put over medium high heat. Add the onion and garlic and sauté until the onion is translucent. Add the red pepper and jalapeño and sauté for an additional 3 to 5 minutes.

4. Lower the heat to medium low and add the tomato, cilantro and lime juice. Simmer for 10 minutes.

5. Add the shrimp and scallops, cover and cook for about 3 minutes or until the shrimp is pink.

6. Stir in the yucca and collard greens puree. Add salt and pepper to taste.

7. This is excellent on its own or over rice.

Serves 6 - 10.

Black Bean Chili

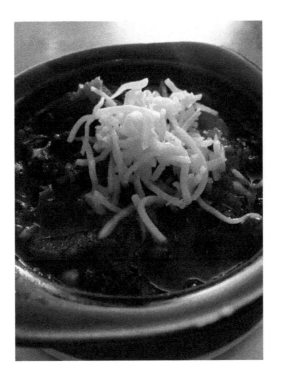

The most effective way to make a plant based chili taste as good—even better—than one made with meat is to create your own chili spice. This is often intimidating to people, but I assure you, it's quite easy and makes a world of difference in your chili. To create umami in your chili with the inclusion of mushrooms!

Ingredients for Chili Spice

You can choose the peppers for your chili according to your own personal tastes and desired heat. I get a combination of dried peppers and often use different peppers with each batch of chili so no two batches are ever the same. (But that's just me) Here are just a few examples.

Chili peppers: Seems obvious to include this classic in your chili. Great heat!

Chipotle: A smoke-dried jalapeño with a smoky flavor.

Cascabel: Small with a rich woodsy flavor.

Chilcostle: Medium heat.

Poblano: milder but full flavored.

Directions

1. Place 4 peppers in a cast iron pan on medium high heat. Make sure the area is well ventilated, (I'd do his outside if possible). Tying a handkerchief over your nose and mouth also reduces the chance of coughing.

2. Allow peppers to roast lightly on each side for about 2 minutes.

3. Remove from pan and place in a bowl to cool. Set outside if the peppers are giving off too much peppery smoke.

4. Continue to do this until you have roasted all the peppers.

5. Remove the seeds from the peppers and chop the pepper skins. Put chopped pepper skins in blender and blend until mostly granulated. Put aside.

Ingredients for chili

1 -pound bag of dried black beans, soaked and cooked overnight OR 4 cans organic black beans, rinsed. Blend 1 can of beans (or 1 cup cooked beans) in the blender until it forms a thick paste.

3 onions, chopped

10 cloves garlic, minced

2 bunches cilantro, de-stemmed, chopped rough

1 cup baby portobello mushrooms, sliced

5 - 8 tomatoes, diced

1/2 cup chili spice mix

2 tablespoons cumin seeds, ground in mortar and pestle

1 tablespoon Himalayan Pink salt

1 teaspoon black pepper

Shredded cheddar cheese (optional)

Directions

1. Sauté onion and garlic in a large pan with oil.

2. Add mushroom slices and sauté until soft.

3. Add tomato, cilantro, chili spices, cumin and 1 teaspoon of salt and pepper.

4. Cook over medium heat for 30 minutes.

5. Add 3 cans rinsed black beans or 3 cups cooked beans and 1 teaspoon of salt.

6. Cook on low heat for 15 minutes.

7. Add bean paste to thicken and 1 teaspoon of salt.

8. Cook over low heat for another 10 minutes, stirring occasionally.

9. Serve and top with cheddar cheese (optional).

Butternut Squash Bisque

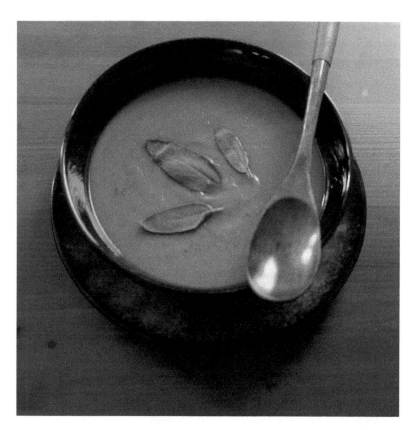

This soup is one of the simplest soups to make and so delicious! Many people like to give their Butternut Squash Bisque a sweet and cinnamonny flavor. I prefer to accent the sweet flavor of this squash with fresh herbs!

Ingredients

2 butternut squash, peeled and cubed

2 medium onions, chopped

5 cloves of garlic, minced

2 sprigs fresh rosemary, de-stemmed, chopped

10 fresh sage leaves, chopped

2 tablespoons olive oil

2 teaspoons Himalayan pink salt

1 teaspoon ground pepper

Directions

1. Add oil to the bottom of a soup pan. Set on medium heat. Add onion and garlic and sauté until translucent. Add herbs. Place squash in the pan and add just enough water to cover the squash. Add salt and pepper and cook until squash is soft (about 20 minutes). Take off heat and let cool for 5 - 10 minutes. Scoop soup mixture in portions into blender and blend until smooth, until all the mixture is pureed. Pour into a soup pan and heat over medium low heat. Salt to taste. Serve warm.

Serves 6 - 8

Creamy Watercress

Did you know that watercress has more vitamin C than oranges? The infamous Captain Cook knew that, and kept watercress on his ships to ward off scurvy.

Ingredients

1 bunch fresh watercress, washed, de-stemmed

1 large Yukon gold potato, peeled, cubed

2 medium onions, chopped

5-7 garlic cloves, minced

2 cups vegetable or chicken stock

1 cup coconut milk

Olive oil

Himalayan pink salt

Pepper

Directions

1. Put 2 tablespoons of olive oil in the bottom of a soup kettle and place the kettle over medium high heat. Add the onion and garlic and sauté until onion is translucent. Add 2 cups of vegetable stock and the cubed potato. Simmer until the potato is soft enough to pierce with a fork.

2. Add the watercress and coconut milk.

3. Add a teaspoon of salt and 1/2 teaspoon of pepper.

4. Lower the heat to medium low, cover and simmer for 10 minutes.

5. Take off the heat and let cool.

6. Scoop into a blender and blend for 30 seconds.

7. Place on the stove again to warm enough to serve.

Notes

Creamy Potato Kale

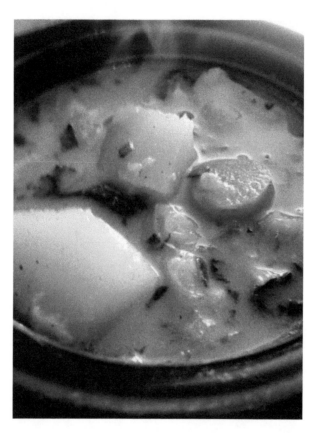

This soup was one of the first soups I introduced at my cafe and it was an instant hit. People could not believe it was vegan because it was so rich, filling, and colorful. Whether you are serving this soup for lunch or at dinner, this special soup will surely satisfy.

Ingredients

3 large Yukon potatoes, peeled and cubed

5 stalks of organic kale, de-stemmed, well chopped

4 carrots, peeled and sliced

1 large sweet onion, chopped

1 cup water or stock

5 cloves fresh garlic, minced

1 bunch fresh thyme, de-stemmed

3 sprigs rosemary, de-stemmed

8 cups coconut milk

Olive oil

1 teaspoon Himalayan Pink Salt

1/2 teaspoon pepper.

Directions

1. Place a large well-oiled skillet over medium high heat and add chopped onion and garlic. Sauté until onion is translucent. Add 1 cup of water or stock. Add herbs, cubed potato and carrot and cook for 5 minutes. Stir continuously. Turn down heat to medium and add the coconut milk, thyme and rosemary. Simmer for 20 minutes. Add chopped kale, salt and pepper. Turn down the heat to low and simmer for more 5 minutes.

2. Serve hot.

Ethiopian Red Lentil Stew

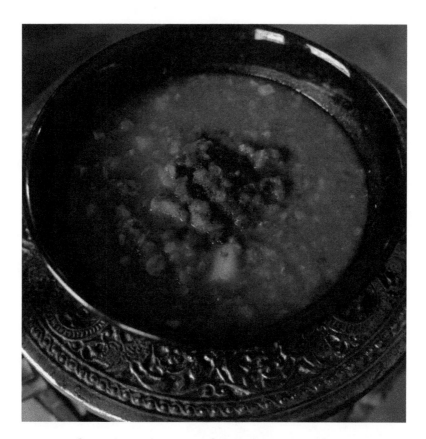

Berbere is an authentic spice combination in Ethiopian foods and is a combination of spices that have been roasted to bring out their unique flavors. Berbere also has some heat! If you love Ethiopian food you love berbere, much like if you love Indian food, you love curry. I have purchased berbere and all of my Ethiopian spice and herb supplies from the website *ethiopianspices.com*. Ethiopian Red Lentil Stew became an instant favorite with my cafe customers and if you like unique spices and a bit of heat, you'll love this stew, too!

Ingredients

1 medium onion, chopped

3 garlic cloves, minced

2 Yukon gold potatoes, peeled and cubed

3 tablespoons Berbere

1 1/2 cups red lentils

1 quart stock of choice or water

2 teaspoons Himalayan Pink salt or sea salt

Olive oil

Directions

1. Place a well-oiled pot over medium high heat. Add chopped onion and garlic, and sauté until the onion is translucent. Add 1 cup of stock or water and the cubed potatoes. Cook for 10 minutes then add the rest of the stock or water and set on medium heat. Add the lentils and salt and cook for another 10 minutes or until the lentils have expanded and the stew is thickening. Stir in the berbere spice and turn the heat down to low. Taste to check the softness of the lentils, and to adjust the salt and level of spice. If you want more heat in your stew, add more berbere. This is a simple, hearty stew and is ready to eat as soon as it is done.

Serves 4 - 6.

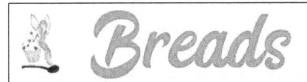

Breaking Bread

Eating meals together has become an old fashioned, quaint idea or something we see in movies from time to time. With cell phone family plans and televisions in every room, 'breaking bread 'with the ones we love has gone from passing the mashed potatoes around the dinner table to sharing fries in the family car. Do we chalk this up as simply our cultural evolution or have we lost something vital in mealtime rituals?

Bread is one of the oldest cooked foods. Every culture has its version and some ritual involving the breaking of bread together. The Ethiopians make Injera, Indians make naan, South American cultures make tortillas, and each European culture has its own signature bread.

I discovered while running my cafe, that the most important part of any sandwich is the bread. A good burger must be put on a good bun or it's just not going to be a satisfying burger.

The griddle naan that I made in my cafe was so popular I often ran out during lunch rush no matter how big of a batch I had made!

Making bread for, and breaking bread with, our loved ones can lift our spirits. The aroma, the taste, and the experience of sharing bread is one of the oldest and most comforting memories throughout human history. We cannot help but feel good when we share freshly baked bread. It is a feeling imbedded deep in our marrow.

Griddle Naan

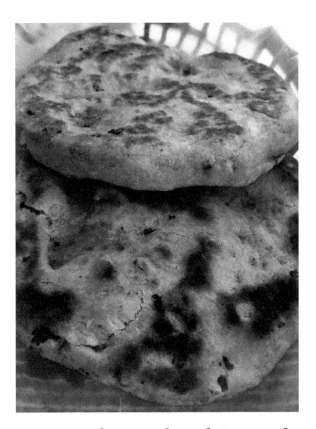

There are many ways to make naan bread. I wanted to create a simple naan I could serve with burgers. My naan became so popular at the cafe, I sometimes ran out of dough in the middle of lunch. But this naan is made with baking powder, not yeast, so I could whip up a batch and have fresh naan on the griddle in no time.

Ingredients

2 cups Greek whole fat yogurt

1/4 cup olive oil

2 sprigs of fresh rosemary, chopped
fine (or your choice of a fresh
herb, like thyme, oregano or
cilantro)

2 cloves fresh garlic, minced

1 tablespoon baking powder

2 cups organic flour

2 cups garbanzo flour

1 teaspoon Himalayan Pink salt

Directions

1. Place the yogurt in a mixing bowl. Add olive oil, rosemary and garlic. Mix well.

2. In a separate bowl, mix the regular flour, garbanzo flour, baking powder and salt together. Slowly add the dry ingredients to the wet ingredients and mix until it becomes a dough. Continue adding flour and mixing the dough until it is thick enough to remove from the bowl and knead on a floured surface.

3. Place the dough in an oiled bowl, cover and place aside for 20 - 30 minutes to let it set.

4. When cooking the naan, rub olive oil on your palms, then roll a small piece of naan in your palm, stretching and flattening it out before placing it on a hot, oiled griddle. Let it brown to your liking on one side, then turn it over.

This naan is delicious for breakfast sandwiches, burgers, and with soup!

Every Day Bread and Burger Buns

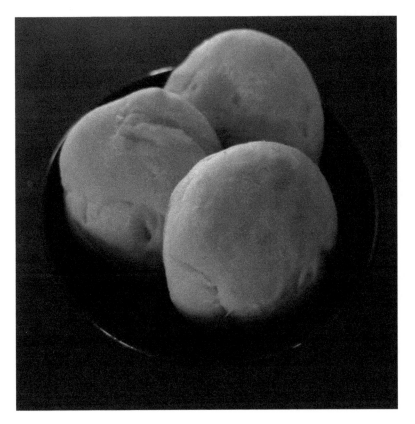

Bread is one of the easiest things to make, yet most folks just pick up a loaf or two from the grocery store every week and never bother to read the nutrition label. We assume the ingredients are simple. After all, bread is a three ingredient food. But if you look at the ingredient list on most loaves of bread, there is a whole paragraph that includes unrecognizable ingredients. Some of those ingredients have been banned in other countries! I'm not going to get into the list of potentially harmful ingredients in common grocery store breads. Honestly, that's your job. I'm going to share a super simple recipe and encourage you to return to the kitchen and try it yourself. I assure you, the bread you make will taste so much better and you will enjoy the benefits of playing with dough (so satisfying), and a house filled with the mood lifting aroma of fresh baked bread. What's not to love about that?

Ingredients

1 packet Fleischmann's yeast

1 cup of warm water (from tap is okay)

Pinch salt

Pinch sugar

3 cups organic flour

1 tablespoon oil of choice

Directions

1. Pour 1 cup of warm water into a medium size bowl. Add 1 packet of yeast. Add a pinch of sugar and a pinch of salt. Let the yeast disolve (about 3 minutes). Stir mixture with a wooden spoon.

2. Slowly stir in flour until the mixture becomes thick enough to remove from the bowl and place on a floured surface. I like to use a whisk at first, then move to a fork as I mix in more flour, then a wooden spoon, until I have a lump of dough I can pick up with my hands.

3. You may need to use a little less or a little more flour to get just the right consistency.

4. Once you have placed the dough on a floured surface, continue to knead it until nothing sticks to your fingers. I like to press down with both hands, then fold the dough and press down again. I repeat this until the dough is smooth and non-sticking.

5. Place the dough in an oiled bowl, cover, and let rise for about 30 minutes.

6. After 30 minutes, remove the dough from the bowl and place on a floured surface. Knead again.

7. Now, if you want to make a loaf of bread, place your dough in a regular sized loaf pan.

8. If you want to make burger buns, cut the dough into palm sized pieces, roll around in the palms of your hands until you have round balls of dough. Place dough balls on an oiled cookie sheet, leaving at least 2 inches between them.

9. Set your oven temperature on 350 degrees.

10. Let your dough loaf or buns rise for another 20 minutes, then bake for 15 - 20 minutes or until your bread turns golden on top.

11. Remove from the oven and let cool for 10 minutes before slicing.

12. Once you see how simple and satisfying it is to make your own bread, I hope you make a habit of it. You can add whatever ingredients you want to flavor your bread. Have fun with it!

Manna Bread

If you know me at all by now you know I love a good story. Especially if it is true! The Essenes were a Jewish sect that lived before and during the time of Christ. They are credited for many of the Dead Sea scrolls. This recipe for a "living" bread—manna—was found in one of them. The key to this bread "living" has to do with allowing the seeds to sprout. The Essenes believed that the energy in un-sprouted seeds is dormant, and the energy of sprouted seeds is alive and thriving.

Though this bread takes a while to make, it is by far one of the best breads I have ever tasted. You can actually feel its "aliveness" in every bite.

Ingredients

1 cup whole spelt

1 cup whole Kamut

1/4 cup olive oil

8 dried figs, chopped (stem removed)

1/2 cup walnuts or pecans, chopped

1 tablespoon Himalayan Pink salt

Warm spring water

Directions

1. Put the Kamut and spelt in a large bowl and fill with water until the Kamut and spelt are completely covered. Cover with plastic wrap and leave on the counter overnight.

2. In the morning check the Kamut and spelt to see if they have begun to sprout. You should see tiny sprouts beginning to emerge from the seeds. If you do not see tiny sprouts, let the it sit out longer. Once the seeds begin to sprout, drain off excess water.

3. Place olive oil, figs, nuts and salt in a large food processor and process for 30 seconds. Slowly add the Kamut and spelt and continue to process. Add a 1/4 cup of warm spring water when you have added all the Kamut and spelt. Within a minute, dough should be present.

4. Take the dough out of the food processor and shape into mini loaves.

5. Place loaves on an oiled baking sheet.

6. Set the oven temperature to 200 degrees.

7. Bake for 3 - 4 hours.

8. The original Essene manna bread was "baked" in the sun.

9. Your manna bread should be crusty on the outside and moist on the inside.

10. Serve warm with butter or with a bowl of soup!

Disappearing Banana Bread

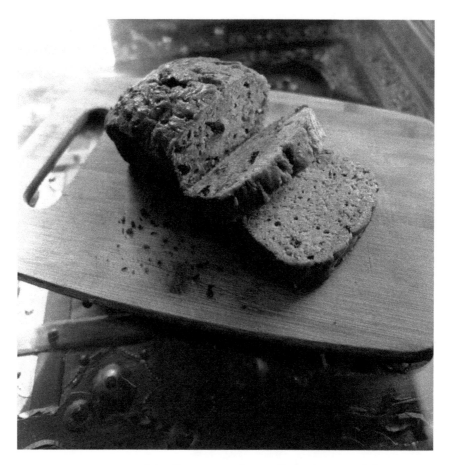

As the name suggests, this banana bread comes with a warning. It disappears! Just this morning I made a loaf, put it on the counter and went about watering some plants on the porch. When I returned, nearly the whole loaf was gone! This can be avoided if one has a good hiding place for their Banana Bread or perhaps a Banana Bread safe for which you alone have the combination. However, this may cause other disturbances in one's home so I always suggest considering the most peaceful solutions.

Ingredients

2 thoroughly ripe bananas

1 cup brown sugar

1/4 cup Crisco (may substitute with butter or olive oil)

1 egg

2 cup flour

1 teaspoon vanilla

1 teaspoon cinnamon

2 teaspoons of baking powder

1/2 teaspoon Himalayan pink salt or sea salt

1/2 cup crushed whole pecans

1 teaspoon butter

Directions

1. Preheat oven to 350 degrees.

2. Place whole pecans on a cutting board and use a roller to crush them into smaller pieces until you have crushed 1/2 cup of pecan pieces. Put aside.

3. Peel bananas and place in a large mixing bowl. Mash up well with a fork or potato masher. Add brown sugar, Crisco, egg, and vanilla. Mix well.

4. In a separate bowl, combine flour, cinnamon, baking powder and salt, and mix.

5. Slowly add dry ingredients to wet ingredients, mixing thoroughly.

6. Mix in crushed pecans

7. Butter the inside of a regular sized loaf pan, thoroughly covering each side and corners.

8. Pour the banana bread batter into the loaf pan.

9. Place in oven and set timer for 45 minutes. At 45 minutes, insert a toothpick into the center of the loaf. If it comes out clean, the banana bread is ready. If it does not, put the banana bread back in the oven for another 10 minutes.

10. Let cool for 5 - 10 minutes. If the banana bread has not disappeared, serve it warm or at room temperature, plain or topped with butter or cream cheese.

Zucchini Bread

I've always thought Zucchini Bread was a wonderful way to get vegetables into our veggie-reluctant children and adults. It also makes for an incredibly moist and tasty sweet bread. There's nothing like a fresh, warm slice of Zucchini Bread with that morning cup of coffee. And it's more nutritious than that donut!

Ingredients

2 cup of shredded zucchini (use a grater for this)

1 cup brown sugar

1/4 cup Crisco (may substitute butter or olive oil)

1 egg

1 teaspoon vanilla

2 cups flour

1 teaspoon cinnamon

2 teaspoons baking powder

1 teaspoon Himalayan Pink salt or sea salt

1/4 cup dark chocolate chips

1/4 cup crushed walnuts or pecans

1/2 teaspoon butter

Directions

1. Preheat oven to 350 degrees.

2. Cut off the stems of 2 small zucchini squashes and shred until you have 2 full cups of shredded zucchini. Place in a large mixing bowl. (Don't discard that

wonderful zucchini juice!) Add sugar, Crisco or alternative, egg and vanilla. Mix well.

3. In a separate bowl, add flour, cinnamon, baking powder and salt, and mix well.

4. Slowly add dry ingredients to wet ingredients, stirring continuously.

5. Put whole walnuts or pecans on a cutting board and, using a roller, crush into smaller pieces until you have a 1/4 cup crushed. Add crushed nuts and chocolate chips to your batter.

6. Butter a large loaf pan, covering all sides and corners.

7. Pour zucchini bread batter into loaf and place on middle shelf of your oven.

8. Bake for 45 minutes, then check the interior by inserting a tooth pick. If the toothpick comes out clean, your zucchini bread is done. If not, put the zucchini bread back in the oven for another 10 minutes or until your toothpick check comes out clean (except for melted chocolate).

9. Let cool for 5 - 10 minutes before cutting. Serve warm or at room temperature.

Notes

Recipes from my Italian Youth

Grandpa and Grandma's Kitchen

Every Sunday after church my father brought us to "Grandpa's house". Grandpa's house was a wonderland of aroma and tastes. He lived with Grandma Lisa, who was not my father's mother, but the woman he had married after Grandma Maria's untimely death. Grandma Lisa was a widow herself, and wore black for the rest of her life, even though she had been remarried.

Neither Grandpa nor Grandma Lisa spoke English. They communicated with gestures and mostly with food. They lived in a little white house with green shutters and rose bushes growing all along a little white picket fence. My favorite place was Grandpa's garden nestled in the back yard, every neat row of rich soil a path through the thick scent of basil, oregano and rosemary. Tomato plants, green beans and peppers supported by wooden stakes, their fruit hanging low and plump.

A young fig tree stood at the center of Grandpa's garden. We thought nothing of the fact that Grandpa had a fig tree in his Massachusetts garden, far from the region fig trees naturally grow. Massachusetts was the wrong climate for fig trees but somehow Grandpa's fig tree matured and gave fruit every year. When the figs were ripening on the branches, we helped ourselves until our mouths turned purple.

One day I noticed a newspaper article in a frame on Grandpa's mantle. In the center of the article stood Grandpa next to his beloved fig tree. I wondered why Grandpa and his fig tree had made it into the Springfield Republican. It turns out what Grandpa had done was close to a miracle. Fig trees don't grow in Massachusetts! The family story goes that Grandpa brought a tiny sprig or the seeds for his tree when he immigrated from Italy. In my imagination I could see him tending to the sapling, covering it in layers of burlap and burying it during the harsh New England months, then bringing it out in the longer and warmer days of spring. What a slow process that must have been! Eventually the fig tree grew to bear fruit in America just as his own eight children had children of their own. I wonder what he thought as he watched us eat the deliciously sweet figs from the tree he had grown from that twig or seed he had carried across the Atlantic in a pocket of his suitcase.

The inside of Grandpa and Grandma's house always smelled like fresh herbs and baking bread. Often on Sundays, when my parents arrived with the five of us, we found their kitchen completely covered in flour. Every flat surface—counter tops, table, chairs—was covered with a sheet of wax paper and flour. And spread across every floured surface was a sea of little hand rolled gnocchi. Tiny little pieces of dough shaped like footballs. Grandma's sauce bubbled on the stove. As intoxicating as that kitchen was, the basement held the most magic and mystery.

No one really knows how Grandpa managed to get a full sized pizza oven into his basement. I remember it was black with chrome handles. Even then, it looked old fashioned. There Grandpa made breads and Sicilian style pizza. To this day, Grandpa's Sicilian style pizza is the best I have ever had.

In this section I have included recipes inspired by my Grandpa and Grandma. Gnocchi, spaghetti sauce, Grandpa's pizza, all inspired by their humble aromatic kitchen and colorful garden.

Hand Rolled Gnocchi

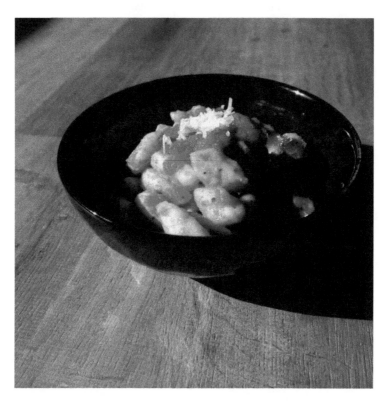

When I was ten years old, I asked that I make gnocchi for my family on a Sunday. I told my mother I wanted to make gnocchi like Grandma and Grandpa, so one Sunday, directly after church, I set about in the kitchen with the task of making enough hand rolled gnocchi for my family of seven. This process took hours and finally every bit of gnocchi dough was rolled out and placed on floured surfaces all over the kitchen. I put the pot of water on the stove, brought it to boil and slowly added all the gnocchi I had so tenderly rolled with my two small hands. I was thrilled to have accomplished such a task. What a triumph! Then, as I began to stir the pot of gnocchi, I noticed to my horror, that all the gnocchi I had added to the boiling water had stuck together in one large gnocchi ball. I remember my younger brother laughing and my mother getting out a box of spaghetti. I had failed. The proud story I had planned to share with Grandpa was ruined.

It would take years for me to learn that failure is an important part of success. I eventually learned how to make gnocchi successfully and to this day am the only member of my family who still makes gnocchi the way Grandma and Grandpa did. I have learned much from kitchen failures and now value them as important learning experiences. When I owned my little cafe, a customer once said, "Everything you make is so perfect." I thanked her but said, "Not everything I make is perfect. I just don't serve you my failures."

Ingredients

6 large Yukon gold potatoes

1 cup whole milk

1/2 stick butter

1/2 cup freshly grated Parmesan cheese

4 cup organic flour

Himalayan Pink salt or sea salt

Pepper

Olive oil

Directions

1. Peel and quarter potatoes. Place a medium sized pot of water over high heat. Add the potato and cook until the potato is soft enough to pierce easily with a fork. Drain and place in a mixing bowl. Add butter, milk, Parmesan, salt and pepper, and mash or mix in an electric mixer until smooth. Slowly add flour until it is possible to knead by hand without dough sticking to fingers. Mix on a floured surface.

2. Roll into pinky finger sized strips. Cut into 1-inch pieces and roll between palms until the dough is the shape of a mini football. Place each gnocchi on a floured surface. Keep hands covered in flour to avoid sticking.

3. Bring a large pot of water to a brisk boil. Add 3 tablespoons of olive oil and 1 teaspoon salt. Slowly add the gnocchi to the boiling water. Stir regularly. When all the gnocchi floats to the surface of the water, the gnocchi is done.

4. Pour the water and gnocchi into a colander and gently rinse with cool water. Put the gnocchi into a pot or bowl and mix with choice of sauce (see recipe for pasta sauce) or olive oil to keep it from sticking together.

5. Serve immediately. Place gnocchi in center of a dish or bowl and top with sauce. Sprinkle freshly grated Parmesan or Romano cheese on top.

Serves 4 - 6

Grandpa's Sicilian Pizza

The best sub and pizza shop in my childhood neighborhood was Giovanni's Pizza in Sixteen Acres, Springfield. I went to Giovanni's for the first time with my friend and first girl crush, Marybeth, and stood at the counter looking at what was labeled "Sicilian Pizza". *That's not Sicilian pizza*, I thought. It certainly wasn't what Grandpa made in his basement pizza oven. These people had gotten it all wrong. Marybeth and I were getting subs anyway, but I never ordered Sicilian pizza from Giovanni's or from any other pizza shop from Massachusetts to New York City to South Florida. As far as I was concerned, Sicilian pizza from any pizza shop could never be as good as his.

Ingredients

Dough

1 packet of yeast

2 cup warm water

2 - 3 cups flour

Pinch sugar

Pinch salt

2 Tablespoons olive oil

Topping

3 ripe garden tomatoes, crushed
   (never from a can)

1/4 cup fresh oregano leaves,
   chopped

1/4 cup fresh basil leaves, chopped

5 cloves fresh garlic, grated

1/4 cup freshly grated Parmesan

1/4 cup freshly grated Romano

1 teaspoon sea salt

Directions

1. When making the dough, follow the directions on a yeast packet. Preheat the oven to 400 degrees. After the dough has risen once, press it down then spread it into an 18 x 12 rectangular pan, and pressing it onto the lip and corners. Using a fork, poke holes in the bottom of the crust. This is to keep it from bubbling up from the pan when you bake it. Place on the top shelf of your oven and bake for 10 minutes. Remove and set aside.

2. Before adding your toppings, brush the crust with olive oil. Cut tomatoes into slices and put slices in a small bowl. Using the back of a spoon, mash up the slices. Add a pinch of salt and set aside. In a small bowl, mix oregano, basil and garlic. Set aside.

3. Grate Parmesan and Romano into a small bowl and mix together.

4. Spread crushed tomato mix on the surface of the pizza dough. Next, add the herb and garlic mix, sprinkling it evenly over the tomato. Next, add the grated cheese evenly.

5. Place on the top shelf of your oven and bake for 15 -20 minutes or until the outer crust begins to brown.

6. Remove from the oven and let cool for 5 minutes before serving.

This is a basic recipe to which you can add topping ingredients of your choice, but you may discover as I did as a child, that the simplest is the best. Enjoy.

Notes

Meatballs

There are so many ways to make meatballs! I am going to share one way of making meatballs but I encourage you to look at this recipe and ask yourself, "How can I use this recipe to create my own signature meatballs?" You can choose your favorite meats. Some prefer turkey or chicken. Some prefer beef, pork or lamb or a combination of meats. Some like spicy, and some like sweet meatballs. It's hard to ruin meatballs, so have fun creating your own!

Ingredients

1 pound ground beef

1 pound Italian sweet sausage
  (preferably without the links)

1 large onion, chopped

5 cloves fresh garlic, minced

1 tablespoon oregano

1 teaspoon thyme

1 teaspoon basil

1/2 cup Italian seasoned bread
  crumbs

1 egg, beaten

1 teaspoon salt

1/2 teaspoon pepper

Directions

1. Preheat oven to 350 degrees.

2. In a large mixing bowl, combine ground meat, onion, garlic, herbs, and bread crumbs, and mix well. Add beaten egg, salt and pepper, and mix together. Form meatballs in the size you prefer,

3. In a well-oiled skillet over medium high heat, sear the meatballs until slightly crispy on the outside.

4. Remove and place on an oiled cookie sheet.

5. Bake in the oven for 20 - 30 minutes or until the internal temperature reaches 160 degrees.

6. Remove from oven and let rest for 10 - 20 minutes before adding to your favorite sauce.

Pasta Sauce

Everyone has their own ideas about pasta sauce. Some are quite content with buying it in a jar. But if you have ever been curious about making your own pasta sauce from scratch, this recipe is for you. Make sure you have all the ingredients before you start! As with most recipes, everyone makes their own version of a sauce recipe once they have learned it. My mother's sauce and my sister's sauce and my grandpa's sauce and my cousin Randy's sauce are all different. I suggest you create your own signature sauce once you learn the basics. Start with this recipe and veer off into any direction you choose. You may want to make it spicier or sweeter, or make it with all pork or all beef or no meat at all. The beauty of making sauce is that you can shape it how you want and it takes on its own unique wonderfulness. Kinda like you. Maybe pasta sauce—not the hokey pokey—is really what it's all about after all. And maybe the secret to everything—love, world peace, the meaning of life—is really in the sauce! All we ever needed to do was get in the kitchen and make some. Happy saucing!

Ingredients

3 tbsp Olive oil

2 large sweet onions, chopped

10 garlic cloves, peeled and minced

2 bell peppers, chopped

1 pound ground beef

1 pound Italian sweet sausage

1 tablespoon dry oregano

1 tablespoon dry basil

1 teaspoon dry rosemary

1 teaspoon fennel

1 cup dry red wine

2 6-ounce cans of Contadina tomato paste

2 15-ounce cans Contadina tomato sauce

Salt and pepper

Directions

1. Place a large well-oiled skillet over medium high heat. Add onion, garlic and bell pepper. Cook until the onion is translucent. Add the ground beef and sweet sausage. (If you have purchased sausage links, cut them into small sections.) Cook until the beef and sausage are thoroughly browned. Turn down heat to medium. Add oregano, basil, rosemary and fennel. Stir in red wine and let simmer for 5 minutes. Add 2 cans tomato paste, filling each empty can with water and adding to the sauce. Stir in tomato paste. Stir in 2 cans of tomato sauce. Add salt and pepper to taste. Cover, turn heat down to low and let simmer or at least 1 hour.

2. Some variations include putting sauce in a slow cooker on low and letting it cook overnight. This produces a richer, darker sauce. Some people, like my mother, like their sauce spicy and so add cayenne. Some people like a sweeter sauce and so will add sugar. You may decide you want more of one herb and less of another, or more or less wine. The fun in making a signature sauce is creating your own unique flavor to share with family and friends.

3. Serve this sauce over your favorite pasta or make pizza with it!

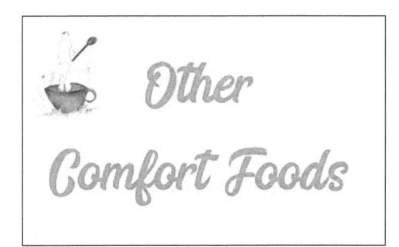

Other
Comfort Foods

Herbed Quiche

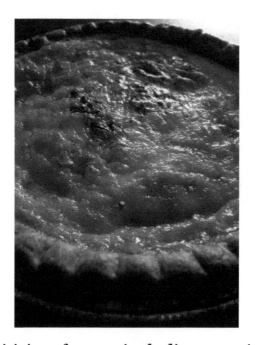

I may get some criticism for not including my pie crust recipe, but honestly, if you had ever stopped by my cafe and enjoyed the herbed quiche, I did not make my own crust. There just wasn't time enough. There are lots of recipes online for making pie crust so if you want to make your own, that's awesome. Just remember it takes a little time to do it right and the crusts that are now available in stores are quite good. For me, the most important places in this recipe to go 'all in'

are the ingredients inside the quiche. Believe me, it's worth it to get the best cheeses for this.

Ingredients

1 pie crust, thawed

5 eggs

1/2 cup whole milk

1/2 cup heavy whipping cream

1/4 cup fresh thyme, chopped

1/4 cup fresh dill, chopped

1/4 cup fresh parsley, chopped

4 ounces Gruyere cheese, shredded

2 ounces fine Swiss cheese, shredded

Pinch of salt

Directions

1. Preheat oven to 375 degrees.

2. Use a fork to poke holes in the bottom and sides of the pie crust. Place pie crust in oven and bake for about 12 minutes. Set aside to cool.

3. In a large mixing bowl, add eggs and beat. Fold in whole milk and heavy cream. Fold in herbs, then cheeses. Add a pinch of salt.

4. Place your cooled crust on a cookie sheet and pour mixture into crust.

5. Bake for 35 - 40 minutes or until a knife can be inserted in the middle and comes out clean. Let quiche rest for 10-20 minutes before serving. Quiche will have "risen" while baking but as it cools, it will settle.

Mediterranean Mac and Cheese

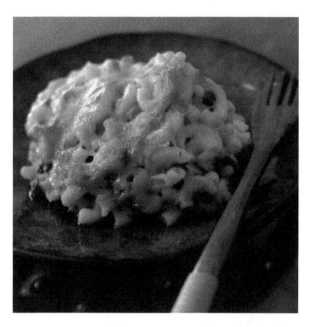

This Mac and Cheese was one of the first signature dishes at my cafe and became a long standing favorite among customers. I have not found another Mac and Cheese with such a flavor combination and could not tell you how in the world I came up with it. I was simply playing in the kitchen. I call this Mediterranean Mac and Cheese because it celebrates the flavors of that region. Mac and Cheese is one of those dishes you can 'customize' to your own tastes. And as with so many other kitchen creations, the best versions of our favorite dishes are often created while playing.

Ingredients

1 small sweet onion, chopped

5 cloves garlic, minced

1/4 cup Fresh oregano, de-stemmed and chopped

2 tomatoes, diced

2 ounces capers, drained

1/2 cup artichoke heart quarters

1/2 cup fresh spinach, chopped

Himalayan pink salt

Pepper

Cheese sauce

4 tablespoons butter

4 ounces cream cheese

1/2 cup shredded Parmesan

1 cup whole milk

3 cups shredded cheddar

1 teaspoon yellow mustard

Pasta

Olive oil

Himalayan pink salt

1 pound elbow macaroni

Directions

1. Fill a large pot 3/4 full and bring to a boil. Add elbow macaroni, a tablespoon of olive oil and teaspoon of salt. Cook for 8 minutes, drain, rinse with cool water, and set aside.

2. Sauté chopped onion and garlic in olive oil over medium heat until translucent. Add diced tomato, capers and artichoke hearts. Simmer on low for 15 minutes. Add chopped spinach and turn off heat. Cover and set aside.

3. Put a non-stick pan over medium heat. Add and melt butter. Add cream cheese and milk, and stir until the cream cheese is melted. Stir in mustard. Slowly add Parmesan and cheddar, and stir until smooth. Take off heat.

4. Fold sautéed vegetables into elbow macaroni. Add cheese mixture and mix well. Put on gloves and hand mix the Mac and cheese mixture.

5. Put mixture into a large baking pan. Sprinkle Parmesan and cheddar, and bake for 30-40 minutes at 350 degrees.

6. Take out of oven and let rest for 5 minutes before serving.

Shepherd's Pie

There are many ways to make shepherd's pie. This recipe is the way I made it at my cafe. Because there are countless variations for meat choices and combinations in Shepherd's Pie, I would suggest using your favorite ground meats. I usually used ground turkey, but this dish is wonderful with combinations that include lamb, pork and venison. It's really up to your personal taste. A satisfying winter dish!

Ingredients

For the Potato layer

6 - 8 peeled medium Yukon gold potatoes

1 cup milk or half and half

1/2 stick butter

1 teaspoon Himalayan pink salt

1 teaspoon pepper

For the meat layer

1 pound organic ground beef or turkey

1 large onion, chopped

4 cloves garlic, minced

10 sprigs of fresh thyme, de-stemmed

10 fresh sage leaves, chopped fine

10 fresh rosemary leaves, chopped fine

Olive oil

Himalayan pink salt

Pepper

For the veggie layer

5 carrots, peeled, sliced

3 corn ears, shaved

1 cup peas

1 cup string beans, cut

1/4 stick butter

Stock from meat and vegetable pot

Directions

1. Boil potato until soft and drain water. Place in a mixing bowl. Add butter, milk, salt and pepper. Mash or mix in an automatic mixer until smooth. Cover and set aside.

2. Put 2 - 3 tablespoons of oil in a large frying pan and set on medium heat. Add onion and garlic, and sauté until translucent. Add beef or turkey and herbs. Add salt and pepper to taste. When the meat is thoroughly cooked, remove from heat. Pour out the stock (liquid in the pan) into a bowl and set aside.

3. Pour the meat and vegetable stock into a small pot, add 1/2 cup water and place over medium heat. Add butter and melt. Add the carrot, corn, peas and string beans and cook until the carrot is soft enough to poke with a fork (but not too soft!). Remove from heat, drain liquid, cover and set aside.

4. In a 1.8-quart baking dish (I recommend Pyrex), layer your pie. The first layer (bottom) is the meat mixture. Spread your meat mixture evenly on the bottom of your pan. Add the second layer, the vegetable mixture, and spread evenly over the meat layer. Spread the mashed potato in an even layer over the top. Sprinkle shredded cheddar over the mashed potato. Bake for 25 minutes at 350 degrees. Remove from oven and let your pan rest for 10 minutes before serving.

(Serves 8 - 10)

Collard Greens with Smoked Turkey Wings

This has been a favorite among friends and family for years and is quite easy to make. Patience is an important ingredient as this dish develops its amazing flavor over time. Letting it simmer all day on the stove over low heat or in a crock pot is perfect.

Ingredients

2 bunches collard greens

1 bunch mustard greens or kale

2 smoked turkey wings

1 large onion, chopped

6 cloves fresh garlic, minced

1/2 cup balsamic vinegar

Himalayan Pink salt to taste

Directions

1. Fill a large pot 3/4 of the way (about 12 - 16 cups) with clean water and place on the stove. Put your turkey wings, chopped onion and garlic in the water, cover and set heat on medium high.

2. Cook for 1 hour, then add the balsamic vinegar and set the heat on medium to continue to cook.

3. De-stem the collard greens, mustard greens and/or kale by holding the larger end of the stem with the fingers of your dominant hand, then pinching the stem where the leaf begins with the fingers of your other hand, and pulling them toward the point of the stem. You should end up with a bare stem in your right hand and a pile of greens. Rough chop the greens, place them in a colander and

clean them well with warm water. Take your time with the cleaning process or you might end up with small grains of sand or dirt in your greens.

4. Cook the turkey wing stock until the meat begins to fall off the bones. Add the greens and stir so they are covered by the stock. Set the burner to medium low, cover and let cook for another hour.

5. When the meat is mostly falling off the bones, remove the bones from the stock, set the burner temp to low. Cook until the greens are tender and full of flavor. Add salt as needed.

6. Serve warm. This dish tastes even better the next day.

Chicken and Pancakes

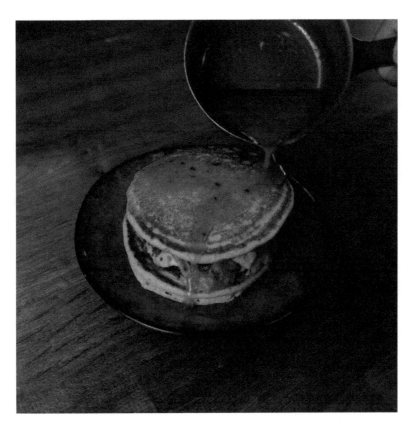

If you have heard of waffles and chicken, it is not such a stretch to consider savory pancakes with a protein like chicken. In fact, pancakes are more filling, and in this recipe, rather than covering them with syrup, we are going full throttle savory and pouring some homemade gravy on top. Game? Let's do this!

Ingredients

Chicken

1 whole chicken(3 - 5 lbs)

1/2 cup fresh sage leaves, chopped

4 cloves fresh garlic, minced

1/2 teaspoon Himalayan pink salt

3 tablespoons butter

2 tablespoons cornstarch

Pancakes

1 1/2 cup all-purpose flour
(preferably organic)

1/4 cup cornmeal

1/4 teaspoon garlic powder

1/4 teaspoon Old Bay seasoning

1 1/2 teaspoons baking powder

1 1/2 teaspoons baking soda

1 teaspoon Himalayan Pink salt or
sea salt

2 1/2 cups buttermilk

2 large eggs, scrambled

3 tablespoons butter, melted

Directions

1. Preheat oven to 350 degrees.

2. Place whole chicken breast up in an oven pan.

3. Mash together the chopped sage, minced garlic, salt and butter until completely blended.

4. Using your fingers, separate the chicken skin from the breast just enough to press small amounts of the butter mix between the skin and meat. Use all the

butter mix, pressing it as far under the skin as you can over the breasts and into the crevices of the legs. Rub a little over the top of the chicken.

5. Cover the chicken with foil and place in the oven.

6. Bake for 45 minutes, then remove the foil and bake for another 10 minutes. Make sure the internal temperature has reached 165 degrees before you remove the chicken from the oven.

7. When the chicken is done, remove from the oven and let sit for 10 minutes.

While the chicken is cooking....

1. In a large mixing bowl, combine all dry ingredients: flour, cornmeal, garlic powder, Old Bay, baking powder, baking soda, and salt. Set aside.

2. In a medium mixing bowl, combine and mix wet ingredients: buttermilk, eggs and melted butter.

3. Slowly add the wet ingredients to the dry ingredients and stir until smooth. Set aside.

Now, for the gravy...

1. Once the chicken has rested for 10 minutes, pour the drippings into a small sauce pan and put over medium heat on the stove.

2. Mix cornstarch with 1/2 cup of water to make a slurry.

3. When the drippings are bubbling up, but not boiling, stir in the slurry.

4. Turn down the heat to low and continue to stir until the drippings thicken into gravy.

5. Cover and set aside.

6. Set an oiled griddle or frying pan on medium heat for the pancakes.

7. Make two pancakes per anticipated serving.

8. To serve, place a pancake on the plate and top with a generous helping of carved chicken.

9. Place another pancake over the chicken and top with gravy.

10. Serve hot!

Notes

Notes

Sauces

Cilantro Sauce

When I began making veggie burgers at my coffee house, I realized I needed to create burger sauces. What I ended up creating were three sauces—Cilantro, Cucumber Dill and Jalapeño Lime—that served as burger sauces as well as dressings for salads. These sauces can be made vegan, paleo or keto.

Ingredients

1 12-ounce jar of mayonnaise or mayo substitute

1 cup fresh cilantro, de-stemmed

1/2 sweet onion, chopped

2 cloves garlic, minced

2 teaspoons yellow mustard

1 tablespoon apple cider vinegar

1/2 teaspoon Himalayan pink salt

1/4 teaspoon pepper

Directions

1. Add all ingredients to a blender or food processor. Blend for 10 seconds, then scrape the sides of the blender or food processor. Blend for another 20 seconds.

2. Pour sauce into empty jar. Pour the surplus into another container and put both in the refrigerator. Let set for 30 minutes before serving.

Cucumber Dill Sauce

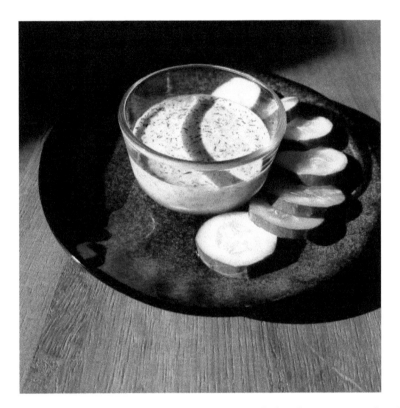

The Cilantro Sauce complimented most of the burgers I had created; but when I created the Falafel Burger, I wanted a different, more complimentary sauce. Tzatziki sauce is so delicious with falafel. I decided to make a vegan version of this sauce for my Falafel Burgers. The Cucumber Dill Sauce turned out to be delicious on so many dishes.

Ingredients

1 12-ounce jar of mayo or your preference of mayo substitute

1/2 onion, chopped

2 cloves garlic, minced

1/2 cucumber, peeled, seeded

1/2 cup fresh dill, de-stemmed

Juice of a lemon

1/2 teaspoon Himalayan pink salt or sea salt

1/4 teaspoon pepper

Directions

1. Add all ingredients to a blender or food processor. Blend for 10 seconds, then scrape the sides of the blender or food processor. Blend for another 20 seconds.

2. Pour sauce into empty jar. Pour the surplus into another container and put both in the refrigerator. Let set for 30 minutes before serving.

3. Use for a burger sauce, on salmon, or as a salad dressing.

Jalapeño Lime Sauce

If you like sauces with a little heat, especially on a veggie burger or meat burger, the Jalapeño Lime Sauce is easy and delicious. Like the other sauces, you can choose your base so it can range from vegan to keto. This sauce is great on burgers (meat and veggie), fish, tacos and eggs.

Ingredients

1 12-ounce jar of mayo or mayo substitute

5 fresh jalapeño peppers, de-seeded and chopped

1/2 onion chopped

2 cloves fresh garlic, minced

Juice of 2 fresh limes

1/2 teaspoon Himalayan Pink Salt or sea salt

1/4 teaspoon pepper

Directions

1. Place all ingredients in a blender or food processor and blend for 10 seconds. Stop and scrape sides of blender or processor so all ingredients get blended. Then blend again for 30 seconds. Pour back into jar and put extra in another container. Cover and place in the refrigerator for 30 minutes before serving.

Raspberry Sauce

I used this Raspberry Sauce recipe for the Brussels Sprout Bisque and for my chocolate mousse, but is also a wonderful flavoring for lemonade and a delicious topping for ice cream.

Ingredients

2 containers fresh raspberries, rinsed

1/2 cup sugar or sugar substitute like monk fruit sweetener

Juice of 1 lime

Pinch of Himalayan pink salt or sea salt

Directions

1. Place all ingredients in blender and blend for 30 seconds.

2. Pour through a sieve into a container to remove tiny seeds.

3. Cover and refrigerate.

4. This sauce stays good for up to 2 weeks in the refrigerator.

Desserts

Sweet Potato Pie

I learned how to make sweet potato pie when I lived in New York City and had just started dating a woman I was quite smitten with. Linda had a sweet tooth and I was determined to impress her with my kitchen skills, and make a pie so full of my affection for her that she could taste it. She did and for years we made a cozy home together in Harlem. A home with a delightfully busy and aromatic kitchen.

Ingredients

2 cup sweet potato, baked and mashed

2 eggs, beaten

1 cup brown sugar

1 1/2 cup heavy cream

1/2 stick butter, melted

1 tablespoon cinnamon

1 teaspoon ground clove

1 teaspoon salt

1 teaspoon ground ginger

1 teaspoon ground cinnamon

Directions

1. Bake 4 sweet potatoes at 350 degrees for 45 minutes or until soft. Let cool and remove skin. Mash.

2. Set oven temperature to 425 degrees

3. Combine sugar, salt, cinnamon, ginger, and ground clove in a small bowl.

4. In a large bowl, combine eggs, sweet potato, and melted butter.

5. Stir in sugar and spice mix.

6. Add cream and mix well.

7. Pour into pie shell.

8. Bake at 425 degrees for 15 minutes, then reduce heat to 350 degrees and bake for an additional 45 - 50 minutes.

9. Remove from oven and let rest for 20 minutes before serving.

Bread Pudding

The best bread pudding I have ever eaten I had at an Irish pub in upper Manhattan and was made with whiskey sauce. This recipe is not made with whiskey and is more kid friendly. I served this particular bread pudding at my cafe and customers really enjoyed it.

Ingredients

2 loaves Italian bread, 2 - 3 days old

2 tablespoons cinnamon

2 cups brown sugar

1 tablespoon vanilla

6 eggs

2 cups heavy cream

1 stick salted butter

1 cup raisins

Directions

1. Preheat oven to 350 degrees.

2. Cut up loaves in 1-inch chunks and place in a large mixing bowl. Add brown sugar and cinnamon, and toss until all the bread chunks are covered.

3. In a separate bowl, beat the eggs then fold in the heavy cream, and add the vanilla.

4. Pour the egg and cream mixture into the bread and mix by hand until all the bread is moist. If the mixture is not fully moist, add more cream.

5. Mix in the raisins.

6. Melt the butter. Let cool for 3 minutes, then pour over bread mixture and mix in.

7. Butter a large baking pan and pour in the mixture.

8. Bake for 45 minutes.

9. Let cool for 10 - 20 minutes and serve with whipped cream or vanilla ice cream.

Vegan Chocolate Mousse

This particular mousse was very popular at my cafe and is extremely easy to make. You do need a good blender because the blender does all the work for you.

Ingredients

4 cups coconut cream*

1 cup sugar (confectioners, regular or monk fruit substitute)

3/4 cup cocoa

1 tablespoon vanilla

Raspberry Sauce (optional)

(See Raspberry Sauce recipe in Sauce section)

Directions

1. The coconut cream is very important here. If you have purchased coconut milk (I highly recommend the brand Parrot), there is an extra step you must do to get the best consistency for your mousse. Place the coconut milk in a glass bowl and put in the refrigerator. The coconut milk will separate, leaving a liquid at the bottom and the semi-solid 'cream 'on the top. Use the cream portion for this recipe and discard the liquid (or put it aside for soups and shakes).

2. Place all ingredients in a blender and blend for 30 seconds. Scrape down sides of blender and blend again for 10 seconds. Pour into a container, cover and place in the refrigerator for at least 30 minutes before serving or until it has the consistency of whipped pudding. Serve plain or with the raspberry sauce from this cookbook.

Notes

Notes

More Fun in the Kitchen

Savory Tallow Candles

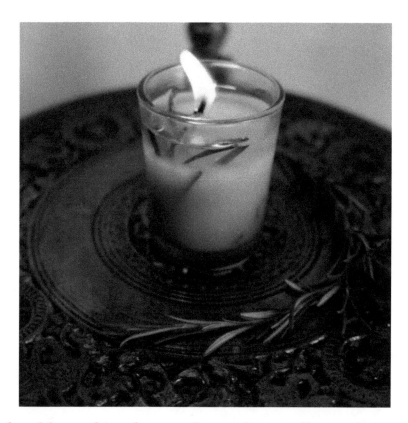

Tallow is beef fat and is what made up the candles and soaps used by pioneers, peasants and farmers before the invention of gas lights in the late 19th Century. Beeswax was expensive and while whale blubber made great candles, not everyone had access to it. When animals were slaughtered, the fat was kept for candle making. The use of tallow candles can be traced back to the Roman Empire. It turns out, tallow and suet have vital nutrients for humans but we have been taught animal fat is only bad for us. This, in my view, is unfortunate. When I decided to make tallow candles, I discovered to my delight that I could get tallow for free from my local grocery store or butcher shop. Tallow (regular beef fat) and suet (the hard fat around beef kidneys) is usually cut away and discarded. I would suggest you ask your local butcher or grocery store meat department if they have any tallow they are discarding. If they look concerned by your request, assure them as I did, that you are not consuming it, but making candles. I even promised the meat department manager I would bring him a candle. I did, of course, and he in turn assured me he would be happy to provide tallow anytime I wished. This recipe includes instructions for how to get candle - ready tallow from the chunks of fat you may be given by your butcher. If you decide, however, not to go that route, tallow can be purchased online.

I infused my candles with fresh herbs like rosemary and thyme. And what a wonderful treat they are at the dinner table! Imagine a candlelight dinner at which you can pour the warm drops from your candle on your meats and vegetables to provide flavor and nutrients!

Ingredients

3 - 4 pounds of tallow from a
   butcher shop or meat market

1 bunch fresh rosemary

1 bunch fresh thyme

Materials

Slow cooker

Cheese cloth

12 3-inch votive glass candles

12 3-inch votive wicks

Wick stickers (non-toxic stickers that adhere your wick mount, and can be bought on line)

Directions

1. Cut the tallow into cubes and place in a slow cooker. Turn slow cooker on high and cover. Let tallow cook for 4 hours, then set at medium heat and let cook over night. In the morning, tallow should be almost all liquid. Turn off slow cooker and let cool for an hour.

2. While tallow is cooling, prepare your candle-making materials. Affix the wicks to the bottom of votives with wick stickers. Place candles on a flat level surface covered with newspaper.

3. Cut 3- inch sprigs of rosemary and thyme and place 2 - 3 in each votive, standing up.

4. Pour the tallow through a cheese cloth into a bowl, discarding any unresolved chunks.

5. Dip a measuring cup or other container with a spout into the liquid and slowly pour liquid tallow into votives. Fill each, leaving 1/2 inch from top. Allow to cool completely. Candles should harden and turn lighter in color. To quicken the process, place on a tray and put in the refrigerator.

Ethiopian Honey Wine

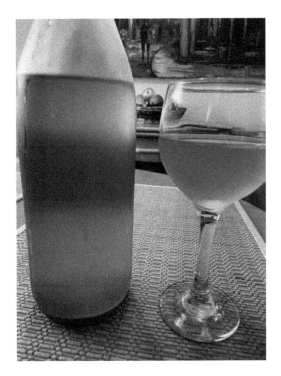

Ethiopian Honey Wine has been compared to mead, which is a kind of honey beer. The Ethiopian wine, known as *tej*, is a unique wine and held in high regard in Ethiopian culture. *Tej* is reserved for special occasions like weddings and is often made specifically for special gatherings. *Tej* is also made with sticks from a plant that only grows Ethiopia. This plant is called gesho and is a kind of hops plant. I have made *tej* for years, usually to give away to special people. It is a joy to find just the right bottles and even design special labels. The very spirit and intention of Ethiopian Honey Wine is celebratory and joyful. If you make this special wine with such intentions, your loved ones are sure to feel it in every sip.

Ingredients

1 gallon of pure water

32 ounces good local honey

2 handfuls of gesho sticks (purchase from Ethiopian vendors)

Materials

1 gallon glass container

Cheese cloth

Funnel

3 - 4 glass bottles with tops or corks

Directions

1. The process of making Ethiopian Honey Wine (*Tej*) takes 5 weeks and is a very simple process. Using a 1 gallon glass container - I prefer a cookie jar container with glass lid - pour 32 ounces of good local honey into the bottom. Add water, leaving an inch or two on top. Stir the water and honey until the honey is completely dissolved in the water. Add the gesho sticks and stir. Cover. (Your cover should not be air tight.)

2. Let sit for a week. You will notice fungus growing. This is good. Stir for 20 seconds and put the lid back on.

3. Let sit for another week. At the end of the second week, remove the gesho sticks, stir, cover.

4. Let sit for another week. Stir for 20 seconds, cover.

5. Let sit for a fourth week. Stir for 20 seconds, cover

6. At the end of the fifth week, the *tej* is ready to be strained.

7. Pour through a cheese cloth. You may do this twice.

8. Using a funnel, pour into bottles and place in the refrigerator.

9. Serve chilled.

Notes

Holiday Liqueur

Nothing says holiday cheer like a homemade eggnog or holiday liqueur. I made this holiday liqueur with all my favorite holiday flavors. It takes just a few weeks to make so if you are serving on Christmas or New Years, make it right after Thanksgiving and it will be perfect!

Ingredients

1 bag fresh cranberries

1 cup raisins

2 apples, cut into wedges

10 cinnamon sticks

1/2 cup cloves

1 small ginger root, peeled, sliced

2 cups sugar

1 bottle of good vodka

Materials

4 12-ounce glass jars with lids

Cheese cloth

Funnel

2 re-purposed wine of liqueur bottles.

Directions

1. Clean your glass jars thoroughly.

2. Fill halfway with cranberries. Add four apple wedges, 1/4 cup raisins, 2 cinnamon sticks, 1 tablespoon of cloves, a few slices of ginger, and 1/2 cup sugar. Fill the jar with vodka, put the cover on tight and shake. Do this with all four jars.

3. Place in a cabinet and let sit for three weeks. Once a week give each jar a shake.

4. At the end of the three weeks, lace a piece of cheese cloth in a funnel and pour the liquid from each jar into a large container with a spout.

5. Pour the liqueur into the wine or liqueur bottles and place in the refrigerator.

6. Serve chilled.

Notes

Homemade Masala Chai

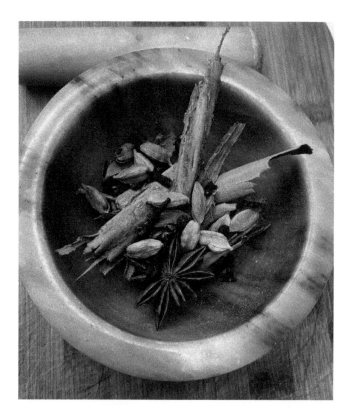

When I first quit coffee, I was at a loss for a morning ritual that would satisfy the morning routine I had so loved for years. It turns out, I was more attached to the ritual than the coffee! When I began to make my own Masala Chai, I became obsessed with this unique process. The whole spices, the mortar and pestle.

If you are dairy free, I would suggest the richest creamer at your disposal (not flavored). And if you are sugar free like me, monk fruit sweetener is a perfect combination. I personally use heavy cream in my chai, so that is what I will list here.

Ingredients

5 whole star anise

2 cinnamon sticks

10 whole clove

5 whole allspice

10 whole peppercorns

Small piece of fresh ginger (optional)

2 tablespoons of high quality Darjeeling

2 tablespoons heavy cream

1 tablespoon monk fruit sweetener

Directions

1. Place star anise, clove, allspice and peppercorns in a mortar and pestle and crush into small pieces.

2. You don't have to grind these spices into powder.

3. Put a small pot on the stove with about 12 - 16 ounces of water and set on high heat.

4. Add crushed spices. Break up and add cinnamon sticks. Add ginger.

5. Add Darjeeling. Stir ingredients.

6. When the mixture comes to a boil, remove from heat and let sit for 5 minutes.

7. Pour into a cup through a strainer. Add desired amount of sweetener and cream.

8. The next time you make this tea, adjust the amounts of the different spices to match your taste.

9. Most importantly, have fun with the process and enjoy the wonderful aroma that fills your kitchen!

Notes

After Dinner with the Crone

The blooms of late summer wildflowers dot the slanted green landscape of the Crone's view. The cooler breezes from the mountains roll across the grass, across the wooden planks of her back porch and across her sandled toes. A scent of clay and the tiniest drops from the nearby stream float along an unseen current. It is dusk and the fireflies have begun to dance in the trees. The sun gathers in golden pools on the mountain tops. Dinner dishes sit in warm soapy water.

She will call Payton tomorrow and thank him again for the two beautiful trout he had brought them. Her Beloved had delicately stuffed the fish with mushrooms and vegetables and served them with roasted zucchini.

"I will make him some zucchini bread tomorrow," the Crone says. "His favorite."

A hand rests softly on hers.

"Shall we walk?" her Beloved asks.

They rise, arm in arm and step onto the worn clay path that leads through wildflowers who tip their purple, yellow and white caps. The fairies stir, the Wee folk glance. A small fluttering line follows the Crone and her Beloved along the path toward the stream. The air grows cooler as the path moves closer to the tree edge and stream, whose silvery laugher rolls and falls over ancient rocks, soothing, lulling the forest toward slumber.

The Crone has a story and her Beloved tilts her head closer to hear. It is a story older than wooden spoons, a story that has weaved through time, across continents and has been told with the gesturing hands of many hues.

A story she has carried in her marrow.

Her Beloved smiles. She knows this story comes from the Great Mother. The Crone will serve it carefully, lovingly in small portions. She will tell it along this red clay path until they arrive home again. She will tell it until her eyes close into sleep, and as the sun rises in the morning. She will tell it over their first cup of tea and later when she cuts garlic and rosemary for their dinner.

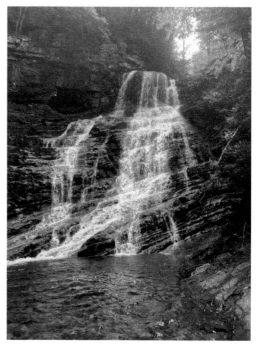

She will tell it to expectant fairies by the fire when night falls again.

This particular story holds a recipe older than all recipes.

The first meal shared between strangers.

Our first taste of humanity.

And this story, the story of the first meal shared in the spirit of our true nature, has been sprinkled like salt on every meal since.

Acknowledgements

This book was made possible with the support of Ashe Rodriguez, my photographer, Taylor Callahan and Bridget Van Otteren, my spirit daughters; and Keahi Elie, my dedicated cafe staff.

Thank you, Ashe Rodriguez, for another wonderful cover and beautiful photos.

Thank you, Kali Browne, for making this book look so beautiful on the inside.

Thank you, Mom, for being such an inspiration in the kitchen.

Thanks to all the loyal customers of Mother Earth Sanctuary Cafe. You made the ten years of our experience a joy.

Thank you to the good people at Larry's Beans Coffee in Raleigh, North Carolina, who supplied me with the best tasting coffee that was also Fair Trade, organic, and consciously harvested, roasted and packaged.

Thank you to Ron Seigal who supplied my amazing teas and took a chance on me when I was just starting out.

Much appreciation to the good people at Don Victorio's Market who supplied the fresh, organic vegetables for my soups and burgers.

Thank you Leprechaun Mike for all your help and support.

Thank you to all the musicians and creatives who graced our tiny stage and filled our space with magic.

A special thanks to (the late) Cleo for your presence, love and support.

Thank you to Hade for being such a healing presence for so many.

Other Books by Patricia Lucia

Wildflowers and Present Tenses (November 2020)

Wildflowers and Present Tenses is the first book in a series of three by Patricia Lucia. Lucia presents the stories in her memoir with a magical twist, creating a Crone narrator, her future self, who tells these stories by a fire to an audience of fairies who gulp up the libation the Crone has left out for them and throw the petals from her wildflowers into the fire - their homage to her. The Crone introduces each story with wisdom and fondness for her younger self. "A woman," she says, "who did not believe she was magical, but held out for magical possibilities."

Coming in 2022

This Amazing Body

A quirky, irreverent chronicling of my personal journey to optimal health in my post menopausal years. Mind, Body and spirit health…weight, sex, food, diet and body image. The bottom line, I've learned, is to listen to our bodies, not the noise from fads, trends, conventional diets, ideologies and cultural expectations.

Follow my discoveries and get some sneak peaks on

Instagram @ This Amazing Body

Facebook @ This Amazing Body

Youtube @ This Amazing Body

Wildflowers and Laughing Crones

Wildflowers and Laughing Crones is the third and final book in the Wildflowers series. The stories center around settling into the joy of aging, the discovery of wisdom, the letting go of unwanted burdens and limitations, the lightening of spirit and the laughter that occupies all the space between.

"I will not go quietly into that great night," says the Crone, "I will go laughing."

Find Lucia's writing, interviews, podcasts and services on

Pattiluciawrites.com

Facebook: @ Patti Lucia Writes

Instagram @ Patti Lucia Writes

Youtube @ Patricia Lucia Author

I would love to hear from you!

patti@pattiluciawrites.com

CPSIA information can be obtained
at www.ICGtesting.com
Printed in the USA
LVHW011058240623
750367LV00065B/890